PRAISE FOR RAISING DOCTORS

"Raising Doctors is an excellent introduction to the world of medical school, a concise but thought-provoking guide for parents."

—*Judy Arnall, bestselling author of "Parenting With Patience and Discipline Without Distress"*

"This easy-to-read, practical, and up-to-date book is on the mark! It is packed full of guidance, wisdom, reflections, and tips for any parent whose child is interested in a career in medicine. Joan Tu is direct, honest, and does not mince words about the preparation and foresight that underscore the challenge of applying to medical school in today's world. The chapters on the stress, and psychological and moral injury, of medical training are essential. Her prose is sincere, warm, and self-disclosing, a big plus. 'Raising Doctors' is written for parents, but it should be read by anyone, irrespective of age, who wants to be a doctor."

—*Michael F Myers, MD. Professor of Clinical Psychiatry. SUNY Downstate Health Sciences University. Brooklyn, NY. Author of "Becoming a Doctors' Doctor: A Memoir."*

"These days, preparing for a future as a physician is often a family affair. This book is a focused, valuable tool specifically written to address the needs of parents wondering how to support their child."

—*Christine Fader, author of "Just What the Doctor Ordered: The Insider's vGuide to Getting into Medical School in Canada"*

Raising
DOCTORS

The Med School Admissions
SUCCESS GUIDE FOR PARENTS
of Future Physicians

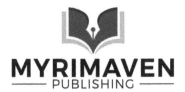

MYRIMAVEN
—— PUBLISHING ——

ISBN: 978-1-7774528-0-3 (print)

ISBN: 978-1-7774528-1-0 (ebook)

Ordering Information:
Special discounts are available on quantity purchases by corporations, associations, and others. For details, contact www.RaisingDoctors.com

DISCLAIMER

The information in this book is provided for general informational purposes only and is not a substitute for independent verification by you (the reader) or professional advice. This book does not contain medical advice. The information provided within is not in any way personalized for you or any reader. The publisher/author provides all information in good faith but assumes no responsibility for errors or omissions in this book. The publisher/author disclaims any liability to you for any loss or damage resulting from using this book or any information presented within.

This book contains links to other websites. The publisher/author does not assume responsibility, and disclaims liability, for any information offered by third-party websites linked through the book or for any transaction between you and any third party.

Raising
DOCTORS

The Med School Admissions
SUCCESS GUIDE FOR PARENTS
of Future Physicians

BY JOAN LEE TU

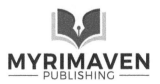

MYRIMAVEN
PUBLISHING

TABLE OF CONTENTS

INTRODUCTION

Do you have a child considering medical school? Have you wondered whether a medical career would be a good fit for your child? An understanding of how applicants get accepted into a medical degree program and become doctors is important to avoid being blindsided by surprises. Without direct and recent experience with medical training, most parents simply cannot anticipate the many particularities and challenges that come with the pursuit of a career in medicine.

Entering the field has changed a great deal in recent years. Traditional science students often, but not always, have an advantage. Even children of physicians struggle to gain admission to medical school.

In fact, it's harder to get into medical school today—in 2021—than it was only a decade ago. According to the Association of American Medical Colleges (AAMC), 53,371 people applied to medical school during the 2019–20 application cycle, an all-time high in the United States, and the rate of acceptance was 41 percent (down from 44 percent in 2010–11).[1] In Canada, less than 14 percent of applicants receive an offer of admission.[2]

This book provides the big picture that many applicants and their parents are missing. It covers what I would want to know if one of my children were to choose medicine as a career. Regardless of whether your child is four, 14, or 24 years old, this book will help to prepare you for your child applying and going to medical school. You will not only see the trees, but also the forest. Without this bird's-eye view, your child could experience overwhelming frustration and disappointment, or waste significant time in their prime years by taking shots in the dark.

Most people simply don't know what makes a strong medical school applicant—or what it actually means to pursue a career in medicine.

This book will help you to:

- *Gain insight into the admissions process, the different stages of medical training, and how long it takes to become a doctor.*

- *Learn what medical schools are looking for—and why competition to get into medical school is increasing.*

- *Learn what credentials, experiences, qualities, and skills your child needs to write an outstanding medical school application.*

- *See how parenting trends may affect applicants.*

- *See why global job and labor market trends and changing medical school admissions criteria are transforming the landscape for medical school applicants.*

- *Gain awareness of difficulties and challenges medical trainees and doctors may face, including wellness issues.*

- *Become a well-informed parent who is ready to help your child decide whether a career in medicine is right for them.*

At the time of writing, I am still a medical student and I have two young children. I wrote this book for parents, to share with you the things that I believe every parent deserves to know about medical school.

What I want most for my own children, however, is for them to have options for purposeful, meaningful work no matter what career they pursue. This book is written in a way to help you support your child in any work they eventually choose.

Autonomy is important in a child's decision to go to medical school. However, if your child truly wants to pursue medicine, they may also need your support in making decisions about their chosen career and their well-being. As the parent, you're most likely the one to make choices about your child's development when they're young and to be the person most concerned with their health over the long term. You have a unique role in raising and caring for a potential doctor.

And doctors, in turn, have a significant responsibility to take care of all of us.

CHAPTER 1:

WHEN MEDICAL SCHOOLS OPEN THEIR DOORS

Some people scoff at the idea that an unemployed stay-at-home mom like me got into medical school. How could it be? Have medical schools become more lax? Can anyone become a medical student and a doctor now?

Quite the contrary; applying to medical school is serious business. Here's how it unfolded for me:

"It's too bad I can't stand the sight of blood, otherwise I would consider medicine." That was me talking to my husband as we went for a walk on our fifth wedding anniversary after a nice dinner.

"That's why you didn't go into medicine?" he asked. "You would just get used to it. That's what I've heard."

"Really?" I wondered. Should I have pursued medicine all along?

"You should look into whether you can apply."

So, I did. I already had the grades that the local medical school was looking for from my previous university degrees as well as a diversity of relevant life experiences. The only thing I needed was an MCAT (Medical College Admission Test) score!

I bought a secondhand MCAT study package the following weekend, and for the next six months, I studied three hours a day, five days a week. I had been a stay-at-home mom for the past few years and was pregnant with my second child. Some days I was too tired, too nauseous, or in too much pain to study. But I just kept going. On the day before the test, I went to see a movie with my husband. I needed to rest and relax for the big day.

That night, my son woke up crying in the middle of the night. Luckily, he went back to bed quickly and I was able to get enough sleep.

I walked into my exam the following morning feeling prepared. In the middle of writing the first section, the test administrator asked me if I wanted a pillow. I was almost nine months' pregnant and I was huge, but I didn't want to be interrupted. I carried on and finished the test even though I couldn't answer all the questions. For some sections, I didn't manage my time well enough to even mark guesses for some of the questions and in the end, left them blank. Darn! I left the exam feeling dejected and deflated.

I had a check-up at the doctor's office that week because I was close to my due date. I had told the doctor about my plans to take the MCAT, and when she asked me how it went, I said I would probably have to take it again as it hadn't gone as well as I'd hoped. But when? It would be so hard to study for it once my baby was born. I had struggled a good deal with my first baby; I didn't want to take on too much with a newborn and a toddler in tow.

Eleven days after I took the MCAT, my daughter was born! I quickly forgot all about the exam. I had a brand new little human being and her older brother to take care of. Some nights it seemed as though the kids would take turns waking up and crying. I felt like I was walking back and forth between their bedrooms all night.

Then my MCAT results came in: I had done well enough to apply to medical school! My score was somewhere in the middle compared to successful applicants at the medical school where I would be applying. I started the process of filling out the online application form, ordering transcripts, asking for references, and locating people who could verify my work and achievements. I was in my mid-30s and was calling employers I had worked for as a teenager.

A few months after submitting my application to the Cumming School of Medicine, I was invited to come in for interviews. The in-

terviews took place over a whole day and when I got home I was exhausted. I had taken all the steps required to apply to medical school. Now all I had to do was wait, but not for long.

On the very first morning that acceptance letters were sent out to applicants, I received my email. "Congratulations!" it said. I was elated. I was going to medical school!

Luckily for me, the admissions process was a relatively straightforward one. Fill out paperwork. Pay fees. Go to school.

As more workers consider changing careers and pursuing medicine, the pool of applicants will become saturated with older candidates who are able to tick off all the checkboxes on the application form before even seeing it. More of these applicants will already have the strong academic credentials and real-world experience that medical schools are looking for.

Dr. Dale Okorodudu, MD, author of *How to Raise a Doctor: Wisdom from Parents Who Did It!*, interviewed 75 parents of doctors and found that over 90 percent had "some knowledge" of what was required to become a doctor, and almost half were "extremely knowledgeable."[3]

As a parent, understanding what it takes to get into medical school in today's world gives your child the advantage they need to be competitive in the admissions process.

CHANGE IS ALREADY HERE

Many seasoned physicians entered the profession under different circumstances than exist now.

Traditionally, medical students have been young, childless university graduates with high GPAs, who completed specific undergraduate courses and hold a bachelor's degree in the sciences.

But you do not necessarily need all of the above characteristics to apply for medical school.

And, times have changed.

THE NEW MCAT

The Medical College Admission Test (MCAT) is for applicants applying to US and Canadian medical schools. In 2015, the MCAT was significantly revised to better reflect the areas that are known to be important for medicine. While "traditional" sciences such as biology, biochemistry, chemistry, and physics are still important areas that are tested on the MCAT, the new MCAT better rewards people who also understand fields like psychology and sociology.

Most people cannot master all four sections (listed in Chapter 2) of the revised 2015 MCAT in a reasonable amount of time, but more people can master at least one, two, or three sections. This has increased the likelihood of success for some non-science applicants, allowing the pool of possible applicants to grow and become more diverse. Yet in 2020, most applicants and matriculants to medical school still come from science backgrounds.

According to the Association of American Medical Colleges (AAMC), of US medical school matriculants, only nine percent came from social sciences backgrounds and four percent came from the humanities in the 2019–20 application cycle, for example, as shown from the table below.[4]

Table 1. 2019–20 US Medical School Applicants and Matriculants by Undergraduate Major

PRIMARY UNDERGRADUATE MAJOR	APPLICANTS	MATRICULANTS	ACCEPTANCE RATE	PERCENT OF MATRICULANTS
Biological Sciences	30,693	12,484	41%	57%
Physical Sciences	4,937	2,355	48%	11%
Specialized Health Sciences	1,964	721	37%	3%
Math and Statistics	344	163	47%	1%
Social Sciences	5,001	1,995	40%	9%
Humanities	1,678	780	46%	4%
Other	8,754	3,371	39%	15%
All Majors	53,371	21,869	41%	100%

MOUNTING COMPETITION

More people from other fields are looking to enter medical school. The reasons for this trend are varied:

- Automation is replacing people with machines in the workplace. Careers in medicine, however, still seem safe. They require people skills, manual dexterity, innovation, human judgment calls, and professional roles that cannot be left up to robots.

- Globalization makes it possible for organizations to cut costs by outsourcing work to people in other countries where the cost of labor is lower than in North America. Much of the work of doctors still requires a physical presence that cannot be outsourced.

- Increased mobility and language skills make it possible for international students and graduates to apply anywhere in the world. Now, instead of competing within a small pond, North American students and workers need to compete with every fish in the ocean.

- Many medical schools no longer require specific undergraduate courses or competitive scores in the sciences. Instead, they value diverse types of achievements, experiences, competencies, and backgrounds.

- Growing numbers of highly-educated students are moving into the field of medicine. These include professional athletes, award-winning researchers, university professors, seasoned physicians assistants, and nurse practitioners, as well as parents and caregivers, many of whom want to undergo a career change.

- Different ideas and evidence related to what makes a good medical student, what makes a good doctor, and the kind of people needed in medicine, are causing medical schools to change admissions requirements.

- Doctors recognize the need to serve marginalized populations who experience discrimination and worse health outcomes than others. Medical schools are making more efforts to help underserved patients by recruiting from their communities and training a workforce that is demographically similar to the patient population.[5]

- Many medical schools have created programs or changed their admissions criteria/processes in ways that address bias and enable more historically underrepresented applicants to get in.

- Many preclinical programs can teach their classroom components remotely and online. This enables them to greatly expand the numbers of students they can enroll and accept more applicants from different cities or countries.

- Jobs that pay a living wage are becoming more scarce, while medical careers still pay relatively well over the long term.

The workers of the next generations are facing a gig economy with more flexible and temporary jobs rather than stable employment. At the same time, millennials already have less wealth than Gen X and baby boomer households did at the same age, partly because millennials have more student debt, according to the Pew Research Center.[6]

Parents are investing more time and resources in raising their children as they recognize this. You may have read about *tiger* or *helicopter* parents or you may have already compared notes with other parents about tutoring, homeschooling, extracurricular programming, or private schools.

None of these trends will reverse anytime soon. Parents won't stop investing in their children, global processes will only become more seamless, automation will continue to displace jobs, and more workers will gravitate to the field of medicine if they can.

IS MEDICINE THE LAST HOLY GRAIL?

Medicine is a noble profession that cares for all people, saves lives, helps the sick, and has a role in improving the health of the most marginalized and vulnerable. Doctors promote and protect health, and preserve humanity in an occupation that is "simultaneously, immensely rewarding, cognitively and emotionally draining, and occasionally physically dangerous," according to Alecs Chochinov, President of the Canadian Association of Emergency Physicians.[7]

The COVID-19 pandemic reminded many of us that the profile of physicians needs to be raised and their voices amplified to advocate for themselves and the people they serve. We *need* doctors.

Given the steady demand for good doctors, and the special and privileged place they have historically held in society, it is no wonder that so many people are flocking to medicine at a time when jobs are disappearing in other sectors.

For me, it was my interest in harm prevention and healing work that led me to discover a particular calling in medicine. Not everyone, however, has a real or clear alignment with medicine as a profession. Many have misconceptions about doctors or do not understand what medical training involves.

GETTING INTO MED SCHOOL IS NOT THE HARD PART

Some people seem to believe that getting into medical school is like winning the lottery: please don't treat it like it is. Don't disrespect the hard work of doctors and medical trainees...and then expect your child to become one!

Medicine is a long-term pursuit and an all-encompassing, life-altering commitment for which medical trainees and doctors make sacrifices to achieve. Getting into medical school is only the beginning of a highly challenging career.

What many people don't know is that every year a proportion of students drop out of medical training—sometimes in the first month—and some doctors leave the profession to do other things within their first few years of practice. Two famous examples of medical graduates who pursued other careers include the late author Michael Crichton and actor Ken Jeong.

Imagine spending years studying to apply to medical school and undergo medical training while amassing a six-figure student loan debt, and then wanting to leave the profession.

Although in these cases all is not necessarily lost, and some medical doctors go on to build successful alternate careers, many applicants and their parents may prefer to not go through the trouble of medical training at all, knowing how frequently this happens. According to Caroline Elton, occupational psychologist and author of Also Human, many "want to quit but feel trapped by the fear of disappointing parents' expectations."[8]

While some new doors to medicine have opened, there are financial barriers, and also medical students and doctors falling through the cracks on the other side. Therefore, medicine is only sustainable as a career to the extent that its members can continue to choose healthy and self-preserving options.

MAKING HEALTHY CHOICES

In your role as parent, think about how you can support your child in developing a career or way of life that optimizes their health. Also consider what you can do to create, or remove barriers to, healthy career options.

There are actions you can take to promote the health and well-being of your child, even if they are already a medical student or doctor. You will know you are on the right track, and well-aligned with the aims of the medical profession, if your actions not only help your child, but also make the world more equitable.

Even small steps can make a difference.

Allow, enable, and help your child to make decisions and incremental changes that align their work with their preferences, and preserve as well as promote their health. Part of the challenge for anyone in achieving a long and successful career is finding the right fit and, rather than feeling trapped by expectations associated with their profession, being able to change course if necessary to continue to do great and interesting things.

PURSUE THE WORK, NOT THE TITLE

Most people associate medicine with doctors who wear white coats and carry stethoscopes, but there are many medical doctors in numerous specialties doing different types of work. The profession requires different kinds of capable people to carry out the challenging yet rewarding work that doctors do. Medicine may need people like your child no matter what degree or career they pursue.

Your child may also work in different areas or occupations over time. Future physicians, for example, will likely be required to retrain frequently and may have multiple careers, according to a Royal College of Physicians and Surgeons Task Force on Artificial Intelligence and Emerging Digital Technologies.[9]

Whether your child wants to save lives, care for people, advance humanity, or make the world a better place, there are many possible avenues available to them and (although not always obvious) most are connected to the work of medicine in some way. Do not fret over having everything perfectly planned out. Focus on helping your child develop the work they find interesting today, and to advance one step at a time.

CHAPTER 2:

HOW PEOPLE BECOME DOCTORS

Let's look at the process of becoming a doctor, what steps are required, and how long it takes.

STEPS TO BECOME A DOCTOR

1. Complete postsecondary studies (minimum two–four years).

2. Look up admissions requirements for medical schools of interest.

3. Take MCAT (3–6 months of study) and/or complete other prerequisites, e.g. tests or courses.

4. Apply to medical schools.

5. Complete medical school (three–four years)/apply to residency in final year.

6. Take licensing exams (during medical school and residency).

7. Complete residency (two–eight years).

8. Apply for fellowship or job.

9. Complete fellowship (minimum one year) or work as a physician if fellowship not required.

Depending on the location and individual medical school requirements, the **exact steps and the order to follow may vary**. The process may also change over time.

COMPLETE POSTSECONDARY STUDIES (MINIMUM TWO–FOUR YEARS)

Medical schools generally require some **full-time years** of postsecondary studies, and most applicants already have at least one four-year degree.

Having a graduate degree such as a master's or PhD can give applicants an advantage in the admissions process at some medical schools, but not always. Acquiring relevant research experience in graduate studies and getting published in scientific journals may be an asset later, however, if applying to a program or specialty that places a high value on previous research and publications.

Some pursue graduate degrees to improve their chances of being accepted into medical school; others finish their PhD before even realizing that they want to apply.

There are universities that offer combined bachelor/medical degree programs; but it's essential to do careful research and consider the pros and cons of these programs before applying. Such programs may have specific requirements or conditions which may not be appropriate for students who need more flexibility.

Some medical schools admit students who have not fully completed a bachelor's degree. For example, applicants who enter medical school after only two or three years of undergraduate studies may prefer to get on with their medical training and potentially become a doctor sooner.

Is there a significant benefit in getting accepted into medical school and entering the workforce as a doctor sooner rather than later? It depends. There may still be a cost to going to medical school early in life, or at the expense of leaving another degree unfinished. Medical degrees are often perceived to be superior to other degrees—which can lead to the belief that a student should not feel bad about giving up another degree for a medical degree. But academic credentials often matter for public jobs in healthcare and in other sectors. For example, some jobs in health administration may require a background in nursing.

For certain roles, having other degrees may still give individuals more options, versatility, and the ability to stand out from other physician job candidates.

Additionally, people of different ages experience medical school differently. I know that I probably wouldn't have succeeded as a medical student in my early twenties. Life and diverse work experiences have helped me to value grit and perseverance. I might have thrown in the towel early and done other things when I was younger.

Of course, that doesn't mean younger students shouldn't apply, or that they should always wait until they complete a bachelor's degree. Many consider themselves fortunate to be accepted into medical school without having to finish another degree, are then successful in their medical training, and go on to become excellent doctors.

But if your child does choose to complete an undergraduate degree—whether or not they plan to embark on a medical degree—the kind of program to pursue depends on their interests and career plan.

PICKING A MAJOR

While some medical schools may still require specific coursework as an admission prerequisite, they allow students to apply after having completed postsecondary studies from all subject areas: sciences, social sciences, nursing, kinesiology, engineering, arts, business, education, or any others.

Students may still want to take prerequisites to show competency and to "cover all their bases," (e.g., through a degree or premedical postbaccalaureate program) 1) so that they can apply to as many medical schools as possible, or 2) to prepare for the MCAT or medical school. But your child should do a thorough review of which medical schools still ask for specific prerequisites before registering for any of them.

Medical schools are increasingly getting rid of their prerequisite courses, usually in the sciences. This trend will be accelerated in the United States as early as 2022 when the USMLE Step 1 (a US licensing requirement that includes the testing of basic science knowledge) becomes a pass/fail exam, instead of being numerically graded. Making this exam pass/fail is in keeping with less emphasis on basic sciences in medical education, unless clinically relevant.

It may be helpful, but not necessary, therefore, for your child to choose a major in an area related to the human body or healthcare such as biology, kinesiology, anatomy, nursing, or pharmacy if pursuing medicine is the plan. It's still possible to pass courses in medical schools without prior knowledge— with a lot of hard work and good time management. Medical students who do have a background in a related field, however, don't need to learn everything for the first time during medical school, which has the advantage of freeing up their time for other activities.

Regardless, grades still matter in the admissions process, so it's important for potential medical school applicants to pick a field of study and a program that interests them—and in which they can excel academically. Applicants should pursue a degree in a field they could potentially thrive in regardless of whether they go to medical school, and not just because they want to go into medicine.

High-achieving applicants and successful medical students can come from all different backgrounds. Saying "study something you're interested in," is more important now than ever, and especially for medical school hopefuls.

Importantly, **grade point average matters more than the subject your child studies, the number of degrees obtained, or the prestige of the university or college they attend.**

In fact, the number of degrees pursued and pedigree of the institution can hurt an applicant's chances of being accepted into medical school if they can't keep their grades up in a demanding program. Studying at a prestigious but academically challenging postsecondary institution, pursuing an ambitious degree program, undertaking heavy course loads, or taking difficult courses that weed out premed students won't be helpful if students can't perform as well as their peers, get lower grades, or lose access to scholarship funds. Such experiences can be devastating for some students, and can happen to anyone.

According to Kirsten Kirby and William M. Kirby, MD, authors of the book *Your White Coat Is Waiting*, pursuing a program that is too difficult is how a premed student's career can end before it even begins.[10]

Finally, with respect to premedical studies, some postsecondary institutions have a premedical committee, and some medical schools (predominantly in the United States) may request a letter of reference from an applicant's committee. This can be advantageous to some students but discouraging to applicants who are refused a letter of recommendation. Before your child enrolls in a program, note whether the institution has a premedical committee and what their role is in supporting premed students in applying to medical school.

You might also find it helpful to locate an experienced advisor (e.g., at a postsecondary institution or via a medical school admissions consultancy) who works well with your child and can help chart your child's course.

LOOK UP ADMISSIONS REQUIREMENTS FOR MEDICAL SCHOOLS OF INTEREST

Medical school admission requirements vary from school to school and may change drastically or abruptly in a single year. So before applying, your child should research requirements to medical schools they would be willing to attend and plan to apply to those schools whose entry criteria match their qualifications.

The Medical School Admissions Requirements (MSAR®) database from the Association of American Medical Colleges (AAMC) is a reliable starting point to learn about admissions requirements at different schools (Canadian universities included). Go to students-residents.aamc.org for the MSAR. If interested in certain schools, applicants should review the schools' websites for requirements, such as reference letters from specific professionals.

I was advised by a physician to apply broadly to as many medical schools as possible, but I only applied to one school. The reason this worked for me is that I had a strong application which matched the admissions requirements for the school that I applied to. There is no sense in your child wasting effort applying to medical schools for which they're a poor fit.

But most applicants should be willing to apply more than once and to go to medical school in another city or even another country. Many applicants won't be a perfect match for the medical school in their city or region, even though medical degree programs often give preference to local students.

Even among applicants who meet all the admissions requirements for their school of choice, competition is fierce, and the majority will not gain admission because other candidates have stronger, more compelling applications. If serious about applying to medical school, your child must aim to make their application as strong as possible.

If additional tests or prerequisite coursework are required, your child should consider the effort needed to complete those tasks and prioritize those which can be done well and in a reasonable amount of time before applying.

STUDYING OFFSHORE

Considering medical school in another country? It's important to do your own careful research.

Studying overseas or in the Caribbean is one way for some applicants to gain easier, faster admission to medical schools. However, be aware that some medical schools have lower rates of degree completion among their students, which may be a concern. It may also cost more to study in another country, resulting in more student debt over the course of your child's training.

It's also a common problem that qualifications obtained in another country aren't always recognized as the equivalent of those achieved domestically. It has been possible, however, for some doctors to practice in Canada or the United States after training abroad.

TAKE MCAT (3-6 MONTHS)

The MCAT is a standardized multiple-choice test that must be completed on a computer at a testing location. Most medical schools require applicants' scores from this test.

The MCAT is administered by the Association of American Medical Colleges (AAMC). As described by the AAMC, there are four sections to the test:

- Biological & Biochemical Foundations of Living Systems
- Chemical & Physical Foundations of Biological Systems
- Psychological, Social, & Biological Foundations of Behavior
- Critical Analysis & Reasoning Skills

Go to students-residents.aamc.org for more information about the MCAT.

Different medical schools evaluate applicants' MCAT scores in different ways in the admissions process, with some schools affording MCAT scores more weight than others in the overall evaluation of an applicant. Different schools also place different value on various sections of the MCAT.

Personally, I recommend taking all sections of the MCAT if applying broadly to many schools. But note that it is not always necessary. I had a classmate who only took one section of the MCAT and was still accepted into medical school. Be aware, however, that this would not reflect well, or even be an option if your child must apply through a medical school application service or later decides to apply to a school requiring scores for all four sections.

To know *whether* and *how* an MCAT score factors into the admissions criteria for a specific medical school, applicants should review the school's website.

WHEN TO TAKE THE MCAT

There is no hard and fast rule for when to take the MCAT. Some students may take it during their second year of postsecondary studies. Others will take it well after they have completed their degree program—up to a few months prior to applying for medical school.

If your child has recently finished studying the material that would be tested on the MCAT in their coursework, and know it well, then it might make sense to prepare for the MCAT right away. On the other hand, your child may wish to wait until they can dedicate more time to study for the test, if needed, in order to achieve their best possible score.

PREPARING FOR THE MCAT

Some applicants will be able to take one or more sections of the MCAT without very much preparation, while others will need to spend a great deal of time and effort studying for the test.

Assuming three hours of study time per day, it takes roughly three to six months to prepare for the MCAT. More or less time may be required, depending on your child.

I studied approximately three hours every day for six months because I had to prepare for all sections from scratch —without having had prior postsecondary training in the majority of the tested subjects.

Different applicants have different strengths and weaknesses. Each person must decide what to prioritize in the study material and determine an appropriate study strategy that will work for them. While some people have great difficulty with Critical Analysis and Reasoning Skills, for example, others can achieve a high score without taking much time to study for this section.

Some students may find certain questions or subject matter to be challenging and should focus on those areas. The MCAT truly is a literacy exam, and it takes time to build literacy in all the different subjects that are tested. Some may even decide on a strategy of picking an answer at random for certain types of questions, so as to have more time to complete the whole test.

Studying for the MCAT takes endurance. Every time I did a practice exam at home, it took a whole day to take the exam and an entire second day to review all my mistakes from the previous day.

Practice tests are imperative for improving test-taking skills and time management. Crucially, they can also highlight areas of strength and weakness, and help students decide what to focus on and prioritize in their studying.

It's important for students to pace themselves, take breaks, get plenty of rest, and not do too much studying at a time.

STUDY MATERIALS AND COURSES

The Association of American Medical Colleges has many resources for MCAT preparation, including practice questions and exams. There is also a wealth of study materials, produced by various MCAT prep companies, to help medical school applicants to study for the exam. Your child should see what is on the market and choose the materials that will help them learn best. It's a matter of preference for the person taking the test.

I compared different study packages and books at my local library. I also read what medical students were recommending on the internet before selecting and buying a previously owned study package that I felt confident about. For me, the look and feel of the books were important. They had to be nicely illustrated and contain summary tables and diagrams to help me visually learn and retain information.

An MCAT preparation course or coaching program may be helpful to some applicants but are supplementary to a disciplined approach to studying. You and your child should weigh the benefits of these programs with their high costs.

It's also possible to learn helpful tips for taking the MCAT by attending free information sessions hosted by the MCAT prep companies, signing up for their email lists, or following them on social media.

And, if the financial cost of taking the MCAT is a concern, check whether any fee-assistance options or free study resources are available.

APPLY TO MEDICAL SCHOOLS

Once your child has completed all the prerequisites necessary to apply to medical school, then it's time to begin the actual application process.

Your child should become an expert in what each medical school they plan to apply to is looking for and obtain all publicly available information from each school about their admissions process. Attending local in-person information sessions is often helpful. If the medical school has an admissions guide, or a video/audio recording about the admissions process, your child should become familiar with it.

Be sure to know the timelines or deadlines for applying to the school. These dates can often be more than a year (i.e., 12–18 months) in advance of starting classes as a medical student.

Some medical schools accept students on a rolling basis (particularly in the United States), such that it's advantageous to apply early in the application cycle, as soon as the application system opens, rather than close to the deadline. Serious applicants must be organized and ensure their applications are complete well in advance.

Medical schools receive numerous incomplete applications every year. These are automatically disqualified from the admissions process.

Medical schools usually require:

- all postsecondary transcripts;
- MCAT scores;
- curriculum vitae and/or written statements (or equivalent);
- reference letters; and
- interviews.

Additional requirements may vary by school.

WRITTEN WORK

Medical schools have firm word count limits, so any personal statements, essays, or any other written work must be tightly scripted. It's not effective for an applicant to whimsically write about what they have done or boast about accomplishments. *Every word* must count toward compelling the admissions committee to reward the applicant with the highest possible score.

Many applicants fail to make the cut simply because they don't know what or how to write.

With that in mind, it's important to have a second set of eyes to review written applications, including personal statements. Rather than only asking for help from personal friends or family members, if possible, your child should ask a medical student who recently gained admission to that medical school to review their written work and provide advice. Or they could seek the help of another qualified person, such as an experienced and credible premedical advisor or admissions expert/consultant.

INTERVIEWS

If your child is invited to an interview, advance preparation is key. I did practice interviews with two different people, one of whom worked in human resources and had professional interviewing experience.

Medical schools interview hundreds of students in a day or weekend. Your child may need to travel to different cities in order to participate.

Some medical schools may require an online test called the Computer-based Assessment for Sampling Personal Characteristics (CASPer®) in addition to, or instead of, in-person interviews.

COMPLETE MEDICAL SCHOOL
(THREE–FOUR YEARS)

Once accepted into medical school, your child might still need to fulfill a number of requirements before the first day of school. These may include:

- finishing an undergraduate degree (if in final year) or current year of studies, and providing proof of completion;
- getting lab tests or vaccines;
- completing a CPR course;
- obtaining a police check; and
- paying tuition, or a portion of it.

Requirements may vary by medical school; your child should follow the school's specific instructions.

PRE-CLERKSHIP AND CLERKSHIP

Medical schools have two parts to their training:

1. Pre-clerkship/preclinical
2. Clerkship

Students spend roughly the first half of medical school in pre-clerkship and the second half in clerkship.

During pre-clerkship, medical students (or pre-clerks) spend most of their time learning in class. In clerkship, students (or clerks), spend most of their time learning in clinics or in hospitals.

Medical students have a set curriculum and learning objectives to complete in order to become what is known as a "physician." Medical schools generally focus on acute or life-threatening conditions that doctors need to deal with, as well as medical conditions that students will commonly see as physicians.

Whether in pre-clerkship or clerkship, medical students must frequently take exams to show mastery of the material being taught. They must also complete OSCEs (Objective Structured Clinical Examination), where they are tested on how well they perform physical exams on patients in a clinical setting.

During clerkship, medical students usually work full days in clinical settings, and then study after hours for ongoing written exams.

The pace of medical school is very fast, and many medical students struggle to keep up—unless they are already well-versed in the material. Even then, medical students often complain of poor work–life balance.

It may feel as though there is always another exam to study for or another assignment to hand in. This is even more pronounced in shorter three-year programs, when medical students train year-round. Unlike those in four-year programs, these students do not take summer breaks.

Often, medical students do not see their friends or family members for extended periods of time. Many even delay starting a family because of the demands of medical training.

Along with exams and assignments, medical students are also evaluated by *preceptors*, experienced physicians who observe students in classrooms or clinical settings. Preceptors hold a lot of power over students during their time at medical school. They provide evaluation scores and comments for the Medical School Performance Report/Evaluation, a report required for a student's application to residency.

APPLYING FOR RESIDENCY

Medical students must complete a residency program to practice as a licensed doctor. As a resident, a medical trainee who has finished medical school works as a junior doctor and receives an entry-level salary. Residents must also meet the requirements and objectives of their residency program.

While in medical school, students undertake career planning and try to identify what specialty they are interested in pursuing for residency. Examples of specialties include family medicine, emergency medicine, psychiatry, pediatrics, internal medicine, anesthesiology, pathology, radiology, public health, dermatology, and surgical specialties, to name a few. Then, in the final year of medical school, students apply for residency programs in the specialties they wish to pursue.

For many medical students, applying for residency is a high-pressure, high-stakes situation.

Even if a medical student is interested in pursuing a certain specialty at a specific location and institution, they may not be accepted for their program of choice. To avoid not having anywhere to go for residency, medical students must, therefore, apply more broadly, either by applying for more specialties or by applying to more locations.

In both Canada and the United States, medical students apply to and rank residency programs, specifying which residency programs they're willing to pursue and their order of preference. The residency programs then specify which students they would accept, producing a maximum of one match per student.

On "match day," medical students find out to which residency program they were matched. Although some students are matched to their preferred choice, many are not, and some students do not get a match at all.

Students are contractually bound to go wherever they are matched. As a result, many students move to another location or train in a specialty that was not their first choice. Some students are unable to stay in the same city as their partner or family.

In recent years, dozens of medical students in Canada and thousands of medical students in the United States have found themselves without a match. Currently in the United States, there is no shortage of students graduating from medical degree programs, but thousands have been unable to secure residency placements to complete their training because of limited funding for residencies. In the main 2020 matching process, 40,084 US medical graduates from MD (doctor of medicine) and DO (doctor of osteopathy) programs competed for 37,256 residency spots.[11]

There are secondary ways for unmatched students to try and secure a spot in residency, but some students still come away without a match. Students who do not get matched may or may not have the option of completing additional training and reapplying.

Unfortunately, there is some stigma associated with not getting matched to a residency program at the end of medical school. And medical students who do not get matched, after exhausting all their options, cannot practice as doctors and may be faced with having to choose a different occupation, despite having accumulated significant student debt. Medical students most often view this situation as undesirable, report negative experiences with not getting matched,[12] and would prefer to match into their preferred specialty.

In Canada, the process of matching to a residency program is administered by the Canadian Resident Matching Service (CaRMS). For more information, go to carms.ca.

In the United States, applicants must apply using the AAMC's Electronic Residency Application Service (ERAS) and matching is done through the National Resident Matching Program (NRMP). For more information, go to nrmp.org.

TAKING LICENSING EXAMS

Medical students are expected to take exams before and after starting their residency to become eligible for licensure.

These exams can be significant for match outcomes or licensure where students plan to practice. For example, in some cases exam results may need to be submitted when applying for residency programs or fellowships.

In Canada, the Medical Council of Canada Qualifying Exams (MCCQE) involve two parts. The first part should be taken in medical school or shortly after graduation. The second part should be taken during residency. For more information, see the Medical Council of Canada website at mcc.ca.

In the United States, medical trainees take the United States Medical Licensing Examination (USMLE) and/or the Comprehensive Osteopathic Medical Licensing Examination (COMLEX). Steps/Levels 1 and 2 should be taken during medical school. Residents should then take Step/Level 3 during residency. For more information, on the USMLE go to usmle.org. For the COMLEX, go to nbome.org.

COMPLETE RESIDENCY (TWO–EIGHT YEARS)

Residency programs vary by location and specialty. Residency programs in Canada and the United States take between two and eight years to complete. Medical students familiarize themselves with the various residency programs and their requirements before they apply through the matching process.

Residents, the most junior doctors, notoriously work around the clock for low per-hour pay. According to one resident survey, "only 34.2 percent of residents report that their work schedule leaves them enough time for their personal and/or family life."[13] However, for some specialties, such as surgery, long hours may be required and even preferred by residents in order to become well trained.[14]

Residents must continue to study and complete required exams for licensure. They also work towards certifications for their specialty.

For more information about certification in Canada, visit:

- The College of Family Physicians of Canada: cfpc.ca
- The Royal College of Physicians and Surgeons of Canada: royalcollege.ca
- Collège des Médecins du Québec: cmq.org

For more information about certification in the United States, visit:

- American Board of Medical Specialties (ABMS): www.abms.org

ENHANCED SKILLS

In Canada, many family medicine residents pursue additional "enhanced skills" training for six to 12 months after completing their two-year residency programs. This training is for family physicians who want to focus on a certain area of medicine or a specific population, such as addictions medicine, care of the elderly, emergency medicine, GP anesthesia, global health, HIV, obstetrics, oncology, palliative care, or sports/exercise medicine.

The College of Family Physicians of Canada recognizes enhanced skills training in some domains with Certificates of Added Competence.

IS A FELLOWSHIP REQUIRED?

For most specialties, a fellowship of at least one year is required after finishing residency. The current trend is that residency programs and fellowships are getting longer and more specialized.

In the past, there were more specialties where physicians could work without fellowships. This is no longer the norm. Even previously less competitive specialties have become very competitive.

WORK AS A PHYSICIAN

If a fellowship is not required, then a physician can find employment or start their own practice.

In the past, a greater percentage of physicians worked in their own practice than they do today. According to the American Medical Association, "2018 marked the first year in which there were fewer physician owners (45.9 percent) than employees (47.4 percent)."[15] Acquisitions and consolidations in healthcare contribute to this trend.

With that in mind, physicians may complete their training and discover they can't find a job in their area of interest. If that's the case, they may choose to work in a related or different role, move to another location, or even to another country to work. Note that more training and exams may be required if a physician moves to a different area of practice.

Doctors must meet the requirements to apply for a license where they want to work as a physician. Sometimes, however, licensure is restricted and not guaranteed, even if a physician meets all necessary requirements. Some jurisdictions have

more stringent and varied eligibility requirements that may
also change with time.

Many US physicians must continue to take exams (e.g., every
10 years) to maintain certifications in their specialties.

ONCE A DOCTOR, NOT ALWAYS A DOCTOR

The process of becoming a doctor is not completely linear for
most medical school applicants. Applicants who don't get
accepted into medical school (or residency) often spend con-
siderable time pursuing other priorities, interests, studies, or
work.

Medical trainees and doctors may also decide to use their
training for other purposes. They could even pursue entirely
different career paths, especially if they can't find work in their
chosen field or decide that it isn't right for them.

With all the excitement and high expectations of family members, it can be an extremely difficult decision for students and
doctors to change course from a highly respected and lucrative
career to pursue a different path.

If your child faces a difficult choice like this, you can ease the
process by making sure you're aware of the challenges of pursuing a career in medicine from the outset. Support your child
in doing what is right for them.

ALLOPATHIC VS. OSTEOPATHIC MEDICINE

All medical schools in Canada and most medical schools in the
United States train in the tradition of allopathic medicine and
are accredited by the Liaison Committee on Medical Education (LCME). Canadian schools are jointly accredited by the
LCME and the Committee on Accreditation of Canadian Medical Schools. Allopathic medical students receive the Doctor of
Medicine (MD) degree upon completion. For more information go to lcme.org.

Approximately 20 percent of medical schools in the United States are osteopathic medical schools accredited by the American Osteopathic Association's Commission on Osteopathic College Accreditation. These schools award the Doctor of Osteopathic Medicine degree (DO) upon completion. For more information go to osteopathic.org.

Applicants to US medical schools trying to decide between allopathic and osteopathic training should research the differences between the two approaches to medicine as well as the long-term career prospects of having one degree versus the other.

In the United States, as of July 2020, osteopathic students must apply to the same pool of residency programs as allopathic students. This is because of a merger between the American Osteopathic Association and the Accreditation Council for Graduate Medical Education accredited residency programs.

While in the past, DO students were able to avoid competing with MD students for residency, the result of this merger of residency programs is that DOs and MDs compete for the same residency spots.

Additionally, even though osteopathic students have their own licensing exams, the COMLEX, all students who wish to apply for a residency program in the United States may consider completing Step 1 of the USMLE to be competitive in the matching process.

CROSS-BORDER CIRCUMSTANCES

While every student's circumstances are different, I have covered the process for Canadian or American students interested in applying to medical school in Canada or the United States *respectively*.

Situations for students from another country who wish to study in Canada or the US are not covered here.

CHAPTER 3:

WHAT MATTERS TO MEDICAL SCHOOLS

So, what makes a good applicant? It's worth your time finding out what medical schools value in their applicants so you can help your child discover and develop important skills and qualities, support their education and career decisions, and plan and parent in a realistic way.

Your child will explore interests and gain life experiences as they grow over the years. They may also acquire the tools they need to be successful in university. But postsecondary studies, and medical school in particular, are not for everyone. Let's examine what medical schools are looking for to determine if pursuing medicine is the right choice for your child.

MERIT, DIVERSITY, AND INSIGHT

Medical schools must balance many priorities when selecting students for admission. Much research has been done to determine what traits make a good doctor and medical student.

After all, doctors and medical students have responsibilities to patients, their profession, and society. They must be willing to both serve and lead others, to effect sound changes where they are needed, and to do the right thing in difficult situations.

They must also be able to withstand the academic and clinical demands of medical training and the medical profession over the long term.

Medical schools look for students who can demonstrate they have the competencies to fulfill these obligations based on what they present about themselves in the application process.

Often, applicants can impress admissions committees based on their merit. Many have accomplishments in certain areas, such as high GPA and MCAT scores, awards, scholarships or grants, publications, presentations, or other accolades.

But medical schools also recognize that many prospective students could potentially spend time at unpaid activities or perform at higher levels because they had more access to resources or opportunities. Perhaps they participated in sports or the performing arts, or volunteered overseas, because their parents had the financial resources and time to support such endeavors.

If medical schools only accept applicants who had access to the most impressive opportunities, the population of doctors gets skewed toward people from families with high financial or social capital. Medical schools recognize that those without power, privilege, or financial means, as well as people from rural or remote areas have historically been underrepresented in their programs.

Recruiting students from underserved communities is one strategy to improve patient care, advocacy, and outcomes for these groups. Because of this, medical schools continue to make efforts to achieve better representation of underserved populations among medical students.[16]

Diverse backgrounds and strengths are needed in the physician workforce to meet healthcare demands. Medical schools are responsible for selecting both diverse and well-deserving applicants who are likely to succeed both in their studies and in their careers as doctors.

Medical schools also place increasing importance on applicants' self-awareness and maturity. Applicants are given the opportunity to communicate and demonstrate self-awareness in their essays and interviews regardless of what work they have done or what they have accomplished. In the medical profession, the word *insight* is loosely used with reference to self-awareness.

Emphasis on applicants' capacity for insight helps level the playing field among those coming from different backgrounds and with varied personal resources. Applicants who demonstrate insight may perform better in admissions processes that reward a combination of merit, competency, and self-awareness.

WHY GRADES AND SCORES MATTER

Traditionally, quantitative academic measures like GPA and MCAT scores have counted for a large portion of the admissions criteria at most medical schools.

Students with a 4.0 GPA and MCAT scores above the 90th percentile were far more likely to secure interviews. This has changed substantially at many medical schools so that these scores count for a smaller proportion of the evaluation for applicants in the admissions process. And today, not everyone with perfect GPA and MCAT scores gets into medical school.

In fact, discussions have taken place about not including GPA or MCAT scores at all in admissions criteria.

But there are a few important reasons why academic merit is still critical for admission to medical school.

1. **Medical schools, as well as professional and regulatory bodies, continue to pass or fail medical trainees and physicians based on their test scores.**

    Medical students must be able to handle a full course load and pass their tests to complete their training. They must be able to work in clinics or hospitals while juggling assignments, planning their careers, taking tests, or preparing for licensure or certification at the same time.

Because of this, they must be highly competent academically, or they risk failing exams and not completing their training.

Medical students who have difficulty passing exams have stressful experiences in medical school. And medical schools are limited in their ability to help such students.

2. **Students who enjoy studying and doing well in school are more likely to enjoy medical school.**

If your child hates preparing for and taking exams, they are likely to be miserable in a profession that requires several years of test-taking as part of their medical training.

A very common attribute of medical students is that many enjoy sitting down to study on a Saturday morning with a pot of tea or coffee. Although there are times when studying isn't the most fun thing to do, if relaxed and well-rested, I thoroughly enjoy my study sessions, learning new material, and mastering the concepts taught.

Many medical students must study, or prepare for class or clinic, almost every day while they are in training. So their GPA and MCAT scores may be indicative of whether your child would thrive in medicine as a profession.

3. **Medical schools are firm on minimum GPA or MCAT score requirements and won't consider applicants who do not meet the stated minimums.**

If your child is interested in applying to medical school, it's important for them to know the minimum GPAs and MCAT scores required by the schools being considered (if they are publicly available).

Applicants with high grades and scores have a better chance of being invited to an interview than applicants who barely meet the minimums. Average grades of medical school applicants are usually much higher than required. For the last few years, at my medical school, roughly half of all new students have had a 4.0 GPA and the vast majority had a GPA higher than 3.5.

Average GPAs of applicants who successfully matriculate into medical school are generally higher in Canada than in the United States, where some students with GPAs in the range of 3.0 may be accepted at some schools.

The MSAR® from the AAMC is a good source of information if you want to find out where your child stands in terms of their grades and MCAT scores relative to other applicants: students-residents.aamc.org

Nevertheless, even if your child doesn't have a strong GPA or MCAT score, it's worthwhile considering schools where they might still be accepted. Admissions committees know that GPAs and MCAT scores are not the whole story.

CONTEXT MAY MATTER TOO

If your child meets the minimum academic requirements, but their grades and scores are lower than most other applicants' they should consider providing some explanation for why their grades were not the best.

For example, if they were working at a job while going to school or studying for the MCAT, or if they had dependents like children or other family members who needed care, where space permits, it may be helpful to write about this on the application.

And, if your child did not take a full course load at some point, or had a particularly difficult term or year, which is reflected in their grades, providing more information about this on their application may be beneficial.

Admissions committees also look at how difficult students' course loads were. They consider where courses were taken—such as online versus traditional postsecondary institutions, how demanding the courses were, and what types of courses the applicant took. They may also evaluate MCAT scores relative to postsecondary grades and courses.

For example, it could be troubling to an admissions committee if a sciences student did not do well on the sciences sections of the MCAT. An explanation should be provided for why this happened. Perhaps extenuating circumstances such as work commitments or family problems made it difficult to study for the MCAT.

Conversely, if a student did not study the sciences in university and was still able to take all sections of the MCAT and achieve a high score, this would be impressive by comparison, which is why some non-science applicants may outshine science majors.

WHAT TO DO ABOUT LOW GRADES AND SCORES

If your child doesn't have an outstanding GPA or MCAT score should they take more classes to raise their grades or retake the MCAT to increase their chances of getting into medical school?

My opinion is to only do so if they can be fairly certain of increasing their GPA or MCAT score substantially or if a higher GPA or MCAT score is needed to meet minimum requirements for medical schools.

Once an applicant meets a school's minimum required score, it is extremely difficult (but still possible) to gain admission only by pursuing further studies or retaking the MCAT. Part of the reason for this is that it takes several years of achieving high grades to raise one's GPA by half a point, such as moving from 3.2 to 3.7.

Many medical schools do not only look at an applicant's highest or last MCAT score; they look at all their scores from every instance the applicant took the test.

Taking the MCAT over and over again without significant increases in scores generally does not reflect well on applicants. Your child should attempt to take the MCAT as few times as possible, only when they feel ready and likely to achieve their highest possible score.

At the same time, grades and scores only make up a portion of the admissions criteria required by many medical schools, and they are becoming an increasingly smaller component in the overall admissions evaluations.

More and more prospective applicants are taking gap years (time away from studies) to gain life experience they would not otherwise have, instead of retaking exams or going straight into another year of school.

Your child's life experiences, competencies, and insight, or being able to express the nature of the work that interests them, all count for an increasingly larger part of medical school eligibility. These characteristics can make a big difference in setting your child apart from others when applying to medical school.

WHO IS YOUR CHILD?

Although not obvious at first glance, there are many layers to this question.

Medical schools require basic facts:

- Name
- Age
- Education
- Awards
- Scholarships
- Grants

- Publications
- Presentations
- Volunteer Experience
- Work Experience
- Extracurricular Activities

But medical schools also ask for much more information than any other typical employer.

The application form for my medical school asked me to list every place I had lived, every school I ever attended, every job I held, every award, scholarship, or grant I received, and everything I had ever published.

I also needed dates, places, and contact information for people who could verify almost every line item on my application form.

Along with every place your child may have made or left a mark, medical schools want to know about life experiences. They want to know what they did or achieved. This may include:

- Academic pursuits including research, teaching, or graduate education
- Clinical work
- Involvement in sports, the arts, or other high-performance activities
- Paid work experience
- Professional activities
- Advocacy and community service work

Medical schools are also interested in *personal* life experiences that have had an impact on your child, which may include adverse life experiences that have been overcome or highly involved time commitments, such as caring for another person or helping with a family business.

These experiences become part of your child's defining narratives. Medical schools may look for ways in which they have shaped your child.

At the most superficial level, these life experiences tell the admissions committee what applicants have done or what has happened to them. But through them, applicants must also effectively convey their competencies.

AWARENESS AND ALIGNMENT

Evaluators should also be able to gain a sense of what has interested your child in the past, and what, therefore, might be an interest they pursue in the future. This includes the type of work applicants would like to do or problems they want to address.

While applicants do not need to know if they want to be a family doctor or a surgeon, or what kind of specialty or population they want to focus on, they should attempt to illustrate the kind of work that provides them with the most meaning, joy, fulfillment, or satisfaction.

For example, some people come alive by creating systems, structures, or masterpieces of some kind, while others prefer to work one-on-one with individuals seeking help or counsel.

Some thrive at solving the world's problems, and others love to teach.

Life experiences also influence the areas and positions in which applicants feel well-aligned, and the issues they want to address, whether advocating for a certain population, or creating an innovative solution for the benefit of all patients.

In many cases, applicants will focus on grades and MCAT scores, undertaking paid or unpaid work that they are *willing* to do, or participating in structured travel experiences that give them exposure to different areas. However, they don't deeply connect to the core of who they are.

Many medical schools now place more emphasis on *meaning-ful* life experiences, competencies, passions, and interests that can be drawn from applicants' *stories* than on academic merit alone.

And although some success stories may seem daunting, because medical students are superstars each in their own way, applicants do not need to have had a wildly successful career or have traveled to the moon and back to get into medical school.

Some of the most interesting medical student stories I have heard were from people who initially pursued careers that did not even require postsecondary studies. After spending time in other jobs, these individuals decided to work toward a university degree, and eventually medicine.

With that in mind, it has become imperative that applicants know or are somehow able to really "find" themselves. Once they do, they can pursue work experiences and roles that are professionally fulfilling or deeply personal.

If applicants are well aligned with their work and continually progress in their activities over a long period of time, they are more likely to achieve flow or mastery in specific areas such that impressive achievements can be made.

Ambitious undertakings, prestigious roles, or a successful career—in ways we traditionally think of success, such as having fame or money—are not necessary to demonstrate qualities like perseverance over a long duration, resilience, self-sufficiency, or self-awareness.

If your child can demonstrate self-awareness, or insight, and has excellent writing skills, they are far more likely to receive a strong evaluation in the admissions process than a person who has simply been "successful." One experience in the context of a person's life can have far more meaning to that person than a similar experience in another person's life.

What an applicant is able to say about their experiences and show in terms of competencies is what compels application reviewers.

PHYSICIAN COMPETENCIES

Different approaches have been used to identify what qualities and capabilities physicians need in order to best care for people as healthcare professionals.

It's well worth reviewing the preprofessional competencies listed on the AAMC website:

- Service orientation
- Social skills
- Cultural competence
- Teamwork
- Oral communication
- Ethical responsibility to self and others
- Reliability and dependability
- Resilience and adaptability
- Capacity for improvement

In addition to these preprofessional competencies, the AAMC website also lists core "thinking and reasoning" and "science" competencies that successful medical students should be able to demonstrate. These can be found at the following website:- students-residents.aamc.org/applying-medical-school/artcle/core-competencies

Many medical schools around the world also look to the widely accepted physician competency CanMEDS Framework of what constitutes a "medical expert" when establishing admissions requirements. You can see the CanMEDS Framework on the Royal College of Physicians and Surgeons of Canada website: www.royalcollege.ca/rcsite/canmeds/canmeds-framework-e.

Applicants who can demonstrate the roles shown in the CanMEDS Framework may be more likely to score higher in evaluations of their life experiences and skills. These roles are:

- Communicator

- Collaborator
- Leader
- Health advocate
- Scholar
- Professional

WRITING WELL

To communicate effectively, applicants must be able to write tightly, making every word count within word limits, while also illustrating the richness and depth of their defining experiences. They must balance vulnerability and grace throughout their written work. I provide further instruction and examples in Chapter 5.

Writing well can powerfully demonstrate strong communication skills and make the difference between a low score and a high score on evaluations of various admissions criteria.

Between two applicants with similar GPAs, MCAT scores, references, and experience, the applicant with superior written work will often be selected for an interview.

Your child must place a high priority on any writing that is part of the application process, and complete written components well in advance of the deadline. That way they have time to solicit helpful feedback and make changes accordingly.

IMPRESSING INTERVIEWERS

If your child is invited to an interview, congratulations! But what do the interviewers expect?

One piece of good advice I received from a physician was this: **What you don't say is as important as what you say.**

Your child should present as "squeaky clean" as humanly possible. Although I do not wish to reinforce intolerant aspects of the culture in medicine, interviewers do judge medical school applicants, and some are more judgmental than others.

Note that the types of questions asked in medical school interviews may differ from the usual job interview questions. Some questions are designed to weed out applicants who may say things that demonstrate a lack of integrity or moral conscience. Other questions may be designed to evaluate the extent to which an applicant has a particular skill or attribute.

Regardless of question type, your child should go through a process of carefully vetting the stories they plan to tell well in advance of the interview.

Medical schools may also incorporate activities like writing, drawing, building, or creating by some other means into interviews. Your child may be asked their position on an ethical question, how they would deal with a certain problem, or to role play a specific situation.

In short, medical schools use a wide variety of evaluations in their interviews. Applicants need to be flexible and adapt to the task presented to them.

Applicants are usually blind to what the interview or question is evaluating, and there is often no "right" answer that would score the most points. Applicants should answer honestly and respectfully in ways true to themselves.

Although this should be obvious to most people, applicants who appear insincere or disrespectful may score lower on interviews.

Medical school interviewers have even seen some applicants curse or rant. Believe it or not, this is why some applicants don't get into medical school! If an applicant is personally dealing with something of concern, poor interview performance may ensue so it's very important for your child to be in the right frame of mind.

Interviewers may not always be physicians; sometimes they'll be other health professionals or volunteers. Speaking negatively of certain professions, workplaces, or former colleagues may not only be offensive to interviewers, but also conveys a lack of respect for workers who are very much essential in healthcare and elsewhere.

Finally, your child should dress in formal business wear for interviews. Suits and dress shoes are standard.

WELL-ROUNDED APPLICANTS WIN

Although academic merit is still important, medical schools also seek to understand who your child is, along with their competencies, potential, passions, and interests.

To convey this, your child needs to be grounded in self-knowledge, and be able to communicate well. This means always having a timely, appropriate, succinct, but well-explained answer to any question that is asked.

Moreover, your child should present in a good-hearted, polished, humble, and respectful manner.

If your child comes from a historically underrepresented/underserved community, it's absolutely worthwhile considering medicine as a possible career, even if they have not had access to every advantage or achieved an outstanding GPA. Diversity and representation are much needed in medicine.

Dr. Danielle Ward, author of *Atypical Premed*, wrote of overcoming her financial situation and low undergraduate GPA (below 2.5) by pursuing an online master's degree.[17] With perseverance and hard work, she got into medical school and became a doctor.

With a strong work ethic and positive attitude, presenting well, and demonstrating insight, your child may very well succeed in the profession.

CHAPTER 4:

SELF EXPLORATION AND DISCOVERY

While your child's situation may be unique and different from mine, I can tell you what prepared *me* for applying to medical school, and what experiences helped me the most in my application.

Classical Greek philosopher Socrates said, "Know thyself." This is where all applicants must start before they even begin writing their medical school applications.

It's not enough for your child to say they are a fourth-year sciences student with strong skills in A, B, or C, who has experience doing X, Y, and Z, and wants to help people. A large proportion of applicants will say something similar in one way or another.

The way to stand out from the crowd is for your child to deeply know who they are and how they are different. It may not be obvious how your child differs from others. There may be significant things about your child that you are not aware of at all.

Children themselves may not fully realize what personal experiences or attributes connect them to others or make them unique. Here are a few things that helped me to "find" myself.

You, your child, or both of you can undertake these activities if you think they could potentially be helpful.

LEARNING THROUGH STORIES

Before I applied to medical school, while I was a stay-at-home mom, I developed an interest in reading the memoirs and personal stories of others. I was searching for purpose, in a sense, because I knew I wouldn't go back to working in a corporate office.

I started exploring trails that others left behind through books and videos. Because I had had personal experiences of violence over the course of my life, I felt connected to storylines in which the authors shared similar unfortunate experiences.

As these stories strongly resonated with me, I gained a sense of how some of the events and circumstances in my life shaped me and still affect me, even today. I also developed an understanding of the breadth of other people's experiences.

I recommend reading memoirs in which people recollect their lives from the *heart*. A story that strikes a chord at the very core of a person is where an answer may lie in terms of their future direction.

The thing about learning from memoirs and deeply personal stories is that everyone gets something a little different from them.

If your child seems lost and not sure what to do, does not know what to write in their application, or is looking for some direction in life, consider suggesting that they try to connect with the personal stories of others. They may discover possible role models and avenues they had not previously considered. But remember, while you may connect with a particular story, your child may not get the same things you did from the books, stories, or films you recommend.

Because I identified with the struggles of people who had lived experiences of violence, I decided to start raising awareness about violence against women and children. First, I crowdsourced children's stories and poems to produce a book, which raised funds for a national charity dedicated to preventing child sexual abuse. I also self-published a second book of my own poems and stories from childhood to raise awareness about violence against women.

In 2016, I began to gather stories of men who had used violence against their partners, but who *chose to change*. I interviewed men about their lived experiences, wrote for a men's blog, and collected stories that were already available in the public realm. I also shared my work at conferences and meetings addressing violence and trauma.

By working for a few years on specific problems in the area of violence prevention, I built a solid network of mentors and peers who support me in this work.

Identifying the issues that were closest to my heart allowed me to:

- Work on problems that mattered to me.
- Find others with similar interests.
- Build community around my work.
- Support others and be supported by others.

By creating this alignment between myself, my work, and the people around me, I was successful in gaining experience, developing skills, and advancing my cause—all of which, I wrote about on my medical school application.

Although it is not necessary to advocate or raise awareness in the same way that I did, if your child finds the core of what matters to them through reading others' stories, it may inspire and propel them to do *something* whether it be research, clinical work, teaching, community service, or helping people in their own unique way.

Different kinds of work that attempt to help people or solve the world's problems are relevant for medical school applications. And you never know; that work could take on a life of its own and flourish in some other magnificent way.

WRITING NARRATIVES

Along with learning through the stories of others, I found another activity that was extremely valuable for my application to medical school: writing out my entire life story.

I spent a few days writing over 10,000 words about everything I could remember over the course of my life.

There were times that I wasn't entirely happy with what I wrote and had to rewrite it. I realized that I didn't really know why certain things happened, or even *what* exactly happened. I discovered that some of the narratives I had assumed about my life were essentially wrong! Certain stories that I always believed about myself weren't entirely true, either because I hadn't had the opportunity or didn't take the time to objectively learn the facts.

As I wrote and rewrote my own story, I eventually arrived at narratives that were entirely grounded in truth. That made it possible for me to share my experiences on my medical school application in a way that was tightly written, objective, and compelling.

In the process, it was especially important for me to write about the worst things that happened in my life, and to also write about things that I was still angry, frustrated, or dissatisfied about. Writing helped me to frame these issues and decide on the best approaches to talk about them—or not talk about them—on my medical school application and in my interview.

If your child is preparing to write a medical school application, writing about adverse experiences can be helpful as an *exercise*, and it's worth encouraging them to do it, *even if these experiences involved you as the parent*. Your child does not have to show you what they write.

If you sense that your child has some unresolved anger or pain, writing may allow them to identify these issues so that they can be appropriately addressed. Being able to get to the core of such adverse experiences, and to graciously and humbly talk about them, should not be taken for granted.

Unresolved problems may weigh your child down or prevent them from speaking in their own authentic voice—until they can find a way to let go of the negativity or emotional loads associated with them.

Reading stories, writing, and discovering one's truth are powerful ways to find peace with the past and move forward.

SEEKING PROFESSIONAL ADVICE

As I worked through some of the things in my past that I didn't feel good about, I saw counselors and therapists. I recommend that anyone writing about personal adverse experiences also seek professional help.

If your child is encountering difficulties, whether in applying to medical school or in other aspects of life, supporting them in both seeking out the right professional support for them and accessing care is vitally important.

Most postsecondary institutions offer or can recommend counseling services for students. If employed, your child may be able to access support through an employee assistance program. Physicians may also be able to provide referrals to psychiatrists if necessary.

Ultimately, it may be best to postpone applying to medical school if your child needs to deal with a current or recent issue. Their health should always come first.

PRIVACY AND PROFESSIONALISM

Give your child the space to freely talk about life experiences that could meaningfully contribute to a medical school application. It may be beneficial for them to receive feedback from an objective third party.

We need to trust our children to do the work and and enable them to speak their truth as professionals. Doctors need the ability to autonomously address their own issues, and to do what is right for the populations they serve. Sometimes that means sharing personal stories.

On my own application, I wrote about the personal connection I had with advocacy projects that raised awareness about violence, and that I wanted to address domestic violence because of my own lived experiences, but I did not talk at length about my personal story.

I chose to focus on what I did to raise awareness and what I learned from the projects I undertook. This highlighted my accomplishments, competencies, and my ability to overcome challenges. I framed my own experiences in the context of my work.

This was the right approach for me, but other approaches may be equally valid and successful for your child.

In the medical profession, there is an ongoing conversation about how physicians and medical trainees can create psychologically and socially safer work spaces. This can be accomplished by exercising vulnerability and sharing personal struggles.

However, there is a time and place for expressing personal thoughts, emotions, and experiences. Medical professionals—including trainees—should still use tact and good judgment in what, when, and where they choose to share. Each individual must decide what is appropriate, depending on the context and on their personal and professional circumstances and relationships.

Some interviewers may choose to probe applicants on their past personal traumas, so knowing one's boundaries can serve applicants well in such situations. In an article entitled "Medical Students Do Not Owe You Their Trauma," one medical student wrote, "questions should be respectful and should not seek more detail than has already been provided."[18]

One thing is certain: a medical school application or interview is not the place to reveal that one has serious unresolved issues or is miserable in some way.

Applicants must learn how to tell their stories with poise, grace, and humility.

EXPERIMENTING WITH TYPOLOGY TESTS

You or your child may have previously taken typology, or personality, tests in the process of career planning at school, or at work. These tests typically assign people to different categories that describe their personality, preferences, or other characteristics about them.

While web-based typology tests, as often used by corporations to collect data, can be controversial, they can also be a fun activity. And they can provide great insights and valuable information to help you and your child.

The most researched, data-driven, scientifically validated typology tests can produce surprisingly accurate results. They not only describe people's preferences in ways that ring true for them, but also give people a language with which to talk about themselves.

Typology tests can provide insights that test-takers may not be aware of about themselves. They can help people identify how they are different and unique.

It was a relief for me to realize that my personality and many of my idiosyncrasies (such as "thinking big" and relentlessly tinkering with a problem to find better/alternative ways to solve it) were well documented and that many people experience life in a similar way to me.

Additionally, some test results offer guidance with respect to career or relationship decisions, advice for dealing with struggles that are common for individual personality types, and a sense of community to people who share similar preferences.

Here are some of the tests I took and how they helped me to understand and talk about myself.

MBTI AND 16PERSONALITIES

One of the best-known personality tests for career planning is called the Myers-Briggs Type Indicator® (MBTI). This test is based on the psychological theory by C.G. Jung and helps people to understand their personalities and make this information about themselves useful in their lives.

Each person who takes the test is assigned one of 16 four-letter acronyms which describes them based on their *preferences*: Extroverted (E) or Introverted (I); Sensing (S) or Intuition (N); Thinking (T) or Feeling (F); and Judging (J) or Perceiving (P). For example, my MBTI result is INTJ (Introverted, Intuition, Thinking, Judging).

For more information about the MBTI® and what each preference indicates, visit myersbriggs.org.

Before I even thought of writing the MCAT or applying to medical school, I did a test online at 16Personalities.com. Like the MBTI®, the 16Personalities test assigns people a similar four-letter acronym, except that Sensing (S) is replaced with Observing (O).

The 16Personalities test described me with great accuracy. Gaining knowledge about my personality helped me to realize that I might be well suited to pursuing a career in medicine.

According to 16Personalities, INTJs like to build things, whether it's systems, solutions, businesses, or even movements. The best careers for INTJs are in engineering/design, research/science, strategy, or medicine.

With that in mind, I had to ask myself: Why did I do a master's degree in linguistics, a domain in which it's difficult to build anything without other skills, and for which there are limited job prospects where I live?

I simply didn't know what was right for me at that time.

If you know and understand your child's personality type and what it means for them you will be in a strong position to support them in navigating life in a way that is well aligned with who they are.

INTJs use their intellect and logic relatively more often than they are warm or nurturing, compared to other people. It's believed that less than 1 percent of women have an INTJ personality. Because it's so rare for a woman to have an INTJ personality, doing the test helped explain why, at times, I've felt misunderstood, judged, or penalized for not being friendly enough or not smiling enough to meet others' expectations of how women should be. I have experienced life as a black sheep in many social environments. Yet I have been successful at many things, including getting into medical school.

Not only was it reassuring, validating, encouraging, and empowering to find out that my personality is well documented, but I also found successful INTJ role models who I could emulate. I found communities of INTJs who I could relate to, and with whom to share common struggles, and brainstorm ideas or solutions that work specifically for my personality type.

INTJs are forward-thinking strategists and contingency plannersA ndrew Yang is a self-confirmed INTJ, while Mark Zuckerberg is often typed as an INTJ entrepreneur.

The truth is that people's gifts usually come at a cost. There is often a trade-off.

Your child's weaknesses may be matched and offset by their strengths. As the parent, by acknowledging this you will be better placed to help your child to do so as well.

Learning about my personality type helped me to embrace my gifts and stop criticizing myself for my inherent weaknesses.

Do you know what your child's gifts are and how to help your child to better utilize them?

No matter what your child's personality type is, knowing more about it may help to:

- Leverage abilities
- Focus on areas of strength
- Develop workarounds for weaknesses
- Identify successful role models with similar personalities to emulate
- Build community

Knowing the results of a personality test may enable your child to optimally align their work, studies, and extracurricular activities with their personality—and, crucially, to feel valued for who they are.

A well-aligned life allows people to be successful in what they do and to navigate life with people who encourage and support them.

And you, as the parent, can possibly better encourage and support your child if you know their personality type. If your relationship is strained, you have the potential to improve your connection by understanding your own personality type and theirs, how your personality types typically interact or clash, and what you can do to overcome any challenges.

Be mindful of focusing on your child's gifts and strengths rather than weaknesses or shortcomings.

No matter what kind of personality your child has, see the positive. Help hone their abilities and learn how to reframe their attributes in a positive light.

For example, perhaps your child gets along with everyone or is good at "working a room" at a networking event. Or perhaps your child is capable of working hard to master or refine a skill, or devising new ways of doing things.

Giving your child opportunities to experience success at what they are good at, or enjoy doing, will ensure they have strong anecdotes and evidence of their abilities for a medical school application.

WHAT SPARKS YOU?

Another typology test I found helpful is the Sparketype test, administered by the Good Life Project. The project was founded by entrepreneur Jonathan Fields, who uses a scientific approach to the question "What sparks you?" The test categorizes people into 10 types and identifies the work that puts people in *flow*.

To try the Sparketype test, go to www.goodlifeproject.com/sparketest.

As I continued my work of raising awareness about violence, I also experienced some frustration because I found myself reading and learning in massive amounts but ultimately having very little to show for it.

I couldn't help but compare myself to others who were cranking out books and blog posts on a regular basis, creating documentaries or YouTube videos, or doing TED Talks. Why wasn't I being more "successful?"

I also wondered if I really would make a good doctor, because there are people out there who are far better than me at nurturing and consoling others on a one-on-one basis.

In society, nurturers are praised—as they should be (but perhaps partly because many caregiving roles largely performed by women are underpaid). As of 2020, nurses have been No. 1 in Gallup's Most Honest and Ethical Professions Poll for 19 years straight.[19] Some people who aren't natural nurturers may feel they don't meet society's expectations of them, especially if they are women or mothers, or if they are in a profession that values the work of nurturing.

I started second-guessing my abilities. If I wasn't nurturing, or "successful," at the work I felt most passionate about, was I good for anything? Would I perform well as a medical professional? Can a logic-driven, not-so-warm INTJ female be a good doctor?

According to the makers of the Sparketype test, *Yes she can!* A person does not have to be all things in their occupation; they can do the work that they are meant to do in many domains and most probably in the domain they have already chosen.

Medicine has many different specialties, each area requiring different work and different approaches. Succeeding in medicine for me is a matter of continually adjusting towards my preferences for work.

The Sparketype test confirmed what I suspected: the work that sparks me is *learning*. Unlike INTJs, people who are "driven to learn" are very common and often serve as subject matter experts. That's exactly what I was in certain domains.

I had created niches for myself by connecting the dots across disparate areas in ways that no one else had. My broad-based knowledge was the foundation for all the projects that I was working on: an infographic, a student organization, articles, and presentations.

Many medical students may in fact be "driven-to-learn" types.

I realized that I could accept and embrace my drive to learn if I became a subject matter expert in medicine and could operate from a position of strength in my knowledge: as a good INTJ, driven-to-learn doctor. These insights increased my confidence in myself and my choice to become a medical doctor, and also reconnected me with the work I truly enjoy.

No matter where my career in medicine goes, I know I must make choices that allow me to focus on the work of learning. When I do so, I arrive at my state of flow much faster, the work gets easier, I feel more fulfilled, and my work is more "successful."

Your child can potentially avoid stress and worry associated with wondering whether they're making the right career decisions if they can discover and then focus on their Sparketype. Being dedicated to their preferred work and getting better at it will enhance their skills, experience, and confidence, which may lead to achievements and impacts not only worthy of a medical school application, but noteworthy in their own right.

Another tool, similar to the Sparketype test, is the O*Net Interest Profiler[20] on a US Department of Labor sponsored website. This self-assessment tool provides actual career suggestions requiring different levels of preparation. It can be found at the following website: www.mynextmove.org/explore/ip

TO KNOW OR NOT TO KNOW

Many people who successfully matriculate into medical school may never undertake this type of self-work. The activities I have described are not by any means essential for medical school applicants. Some find their true selves in other ways, perhaps by having the support to pursue opportunities and interests, or joining communities with which they identify, without reading or writing memoirs, or taking personality tests.

Others have such impressive credentials, grades, and scores that they can already do well—compared to other candidates—when their applications are evaluated.

Yet as competition increases, more applicants will present with uniformly good grades and scores, and impressive achievements from having created alignment between their stories, their strengths, and their work. Without first knowing and embracing their gifts, however, it will be more difficult for applicants to gain admission to medical school. With the help of narratives or typology tests, you can support and encourage your child in pursuits that are authentic and aligned well to them.

This alignment and self-knowledge will help them in later career stages including medical training, while practicing as a doctor, or even pursuing an entirely different profession. In the book *Your White Coat Is Waiting*, Dr. William Kirby recommends that applicants know themselves so that they can become strong advocates for themselves and can more aggres-

sively seek out situations that fit their abilities and personality.[21]

Of course, every person is different. Your child may not want
to be labeled with types and categories or for you to know
or apply theories about them. Be wary of over-applying any
knowledge you gain from these exercises.

If your child has no interest in them, you can still pursue these
activities for yourself. You may benefit from going through a
similar process of knowing yourself better and this process can
help produce positive ripple effects, which may also benefit
your child.

CHAPTER 5:

APPLYING TO MEDICAL SCHOOL

As noted, writing a strong application and performing well at the interview are both critical in the process of applying to medical school.

With that in mind, here is how I approached the task of writing my own medical school application, including samples of what I wrote, and some insights from my experience of the interview process.

TACKLING WRITTEN WORK

When we introduce ourselves to others, most of the time we talk about or present our most outer layers. We usually tell people how they may refer to us and what we do. For example, "I'm a mom. I have two little kids. They're three and six years old. I'm also a medical student. My husband is an engineer."

Another example might sound like this: "I'm a fourth-year biology student. Over the summer, I helped a professor with a research project. I learned how to collect and analyze data and write a paper. My parents didn't have very much when I was growing up. I helped my brother a lot because of his illness. I run every day to stay healthy. Last year I ran a marathon."

All of this is fine to say, but in a medical school application, applicants must go layers deeper.

No one would argue that many of the accomplishments and identifiers described above show dedication, hard work, perseverance, willpower, or the desire to do well. With reference to the above descriptions, we can most likely agree that:

- Parents, caregivers, and medical students are hard-working. Being a parent and medical student at the same time is difficult.
- Becoming and working as an engineer takes time and persistence.
- Studying biology and doing research is important work.
- Working at a job requires a strong work ethic, the habit of showing up every day, and doing good work.
- Learning and honing skills takes initiative, practice, and continuous improvement.
- It's challenging and unfair to experience poverty or the adverse effects of a chronic health problem; dealing with these conditions demonstrates resilience.
- Running and prioritizing health show self-care and balance.
- Running a marathon is goal-oriented, ambitious, and takes hard work!

But it is not enough to write like this on a medical school application. **Applicants must write about their experiences, skills, attributes, and work in a way that is as unique as their fingerprint.**

What insights can your child share about who they are, what they have done, or what has happened in their lives that make these things truly and only theirs?

Instead of writing paragraphs of *lists*, they must write paragraphs of *stories*. There is no need to state or describe most experiences, skills, attributes, or work preferences if they can demonstrate these things in their stories.

In other words: **Show, don't tell.**

Your child may wish to consider the following questions about their relevant experiences while considering what to say on a medical school application:

- What went well? Why?
- What did not go so well? Why?
- What was challenging for you? What did you struggle with? How did you address or overcome this?
- Would you have changed anything? What would you have changed?
- What specific mistakes or failures did you learn from? What did you learn?
- Are there any experiences, people, moments, or lessons that made an impact on you? In what way?
- What are your most important/meaningful accomplishments or proudest moments? Why?

All these questions will force an applicant to tell a story that describes a deeper, more unique insight than simply sharing a fact.

Ultimately, **applicants must be able to tell stories that portray themselves in a positive light.**

Here are some example paragraphs from my own application.

I managed a team of eight students in organizing numerous events/fundraisers and deciding on the allocation of funds to enhance the student experience and support important causes. I was also an ambassador for the school at events such as Open Houses.

Looking back, I was fortunate to have team members who executed our plans successfully. It was my first truly challenging leadership experience. Although I was elected onto the Student Council by students, it was the advisor (a teacher) who selected me to be President. I gained exposure to what it is like to have my leadership frequently questioned. A couple of people on my team insisted we do things that I felt were outside the scope of our role (such as get involved in politics outside of the school or organize a rave at school).

In retrospect, I wish I had consulted the advisor for guidance when I encountered these questions about the scope of my role and had asked for help. I learned about setting expectations/delegating when student volunteers abandoned their shifts at coat check and coats were lost/stolen at that school dance. One of them later said we should have hired a coat-check service. I grew into the role, however, and was encouraged to take on future leadership roles.

In this case, I held the title of student council president, but it isn't necessary to hold roles with official or important titles to apply to medical school. It's better if your child writes about experiences or work that they have a lot to say about, than to write about a role that came with an impressive title, but that didn't require very much of them.

From my example paragraphs, you can see that your child should try to do the following:

- Briefly describe a role in terms of its function and scope. (If particularly proud of an accomplishment, mention it.)

- Make every word count. Use short but meaningful sentences to convey perspectives about the experience. (For example, instead of saying, "This happened 17 years ago. I'm a much older and wiser person now, and I'm only going to describe this experience in broad strokes," I started with, "Looking back.")

- Convey a sense of the emotions associated with the experience. (Instead of writing about all the activities that my team accomplished, I expressed my gratitude and the impression that the experience left with me by saying, "I was fortunate to have team members who executed our plans successfully.")

- Highlight positive personal attributes. (My example demonstrated that I had some broad-based support from students, and that there was also something dependable about me that a teacher could trust in choosing me to be student council president.)

- Illustrate challenges. (I talked about how hard it was to hold a leadership position and how I didn't know how to deal with new challenges at first.)
- Share lessons learned. (I described how things didn't go as I expected or as I had planned, and how I came to recognize the importance of asking for help.)
- Summarize the outcome and put the experience into context. (I said "I grew into the role" because I didn't give up! I did the job. I was capable of being president of my student council. I even took on other leadership positions after high school.)

While I've done a lot of explaining here about what I wrote, I didn't need to do that in my actual application because stories are loaded with information if they are written in a way that captures the intended nuances.

Applicants don't necessarily have to list everything that they have done or that they are, or to make generic statements like, "I was able to learn from my mistakes." This type of information should come across in the story to avoid wasting words or space.

Another writing sample from my application reads as follows:

From 2000 to 2004, I took on increasingly challenging roles as a volunteer for AIESEC, an international student organization. In 2005, I completed an international work exchange at Tertia Edusoft facilitated by AIESEC in Germany.

As President of AIESEC in Calgary I managed a team of seven executives among a membership of 50 volunteers who ran an international work exchange program and organized events (e.g., careers day). I trained/mentored dozens of student volunteers. As VP Exchange, I recruited/screened applicants, helped students obtain international work placements, and facilitated preparation sessions about culture shock/working abroad. I gained insights into diverse cultures, beliefs, and paradigms through friendships with people from different countries. My parents were first-generation immigrants, so I appreciated AIESEC's values of embracing diver-

sity/world peace as well as the opportunity to live/work abroad. At Tertia Edusoft, I rewrote English user manuals. I learned about Germany and its people through my workplace, interactions with AIESEC members, German classes, and by meeting with multiple language exchange partners every week. I learned enough German to translate from German to English.

These paragraphs highlight different experiences and attributes than my first example and prove that I took on additional leadership roles in university.

In my case I demonstrated continuity of leadership experience, but research, advocacy, community service, clinical, or other activities are just as, if not more, valuable.

What the reader can see from these paragraphs is that I actually did a *lot of stuff* over time. I stayed with this one organization for a few years, gained skills and experience in it, progressively used my competencies in different capacities, and advanced into more challenging roles.

If I had been a much younger applicant, I could have written more about my involvement with AIESEC and had separate paragraphs for different roles I held in the organization. I condensed it all into one paragraph, however, because I still had to write about activities and experiences that happened later in my life.

From what I wrote, you can see how your child should:

- Show rather than tell. (It isn't necessary to explicitly say, "I stuck with this group for a long time," or to make general statements like, "I am an organized, competent, highly motivated individual," if you can show it through a story.)
- Make personal connections. (In my example, I do this by talking about the friendships I made, how I learned about different cultures and ideas, and how I was exposed to working in another country in relation to my parents' experience as immigrants.)

Here's a final example from my application, in which I talk about my experience working as a debt counselor.

I gained experience working with a diverse clientele (including vulnerable/marginalized populations) and gained exposure to a wide variety of financial problems that people encounter for many different reasons. I became familiar with services/resources for those in financial need/distress. I came to recognize that some options which seemed unfavorable to me are valid options for certain people/situations. I became more open-minded about the various options available to resolve financial issues. I was frequently given honest/helpful feedback as part of the on-the-job training. I realized that I wanted to be more like the experienced counselors (both personally and professionally) in being able to assertively give constructive feedback and help people. One day I was told that I was not hearing what the client wanted. I realized that I could become more self-aware in order to prevent my beliefs/biases from hindering my ability to listen to clients and respect what they actually want.

This example shows that I worked in a counseling capacity; in this case, helping people with money rather than health problems. I saw a different side of people that most people don't ever see and could bring the insights I gained about those problems and solutions to my work in medicine.

The paragraph also shows that I was *coachable*. I saw the good in others and how they were better at some things than I was. I valued the feedback I was given and internalized it, in a role where I was not a leader.

I had to write several paragraphs like these in preparing my application. I even wrote a paragraph about parenthood.

In every sentence of their application, your child should aim to:

- Say as much as possible that has not been said anywhere else in the application.
- Omit anything that isn't necessary to say because it will come across anyway.

- Demonstrate what the experiences *meant* rather than just what they were.

If your child is struggling with what to write or whether they can write effectively, it may be worthwhile engaging an expert who specializes in medical school applications who can advise your child.

Written sections of a medical school application can make or break a person's chances of securing an interview. Many applicants have excellent grades and experience, but they do not get interviews because they do not effectively communicate in their writing.

What or how applicants write may also count towards any evaluations or scores related to communication skills. Having a tightly written application that shows merit, depth, and insight, demonstrates both masterful communication skills and the self-awareness that medical schools are looking for.

To summarize, your child's medical school application should:

- Briefly describe roles and accomplishments.
- Make every word count.
- Convey a sense of the emotions associated with the experience.
- Highlight positive personal attributes.
- Illustrate challenges.
- Share lessons learned.
- Summarize outcomes.
- Put experiences into context.
- Show, don't tell.
- Make personal connections.

Early readers of this book, said the above section would be particularly helpful to applicants so I have adapted it as a standalone guide called "How to Write Personal Narratives for Medical School Applications," available at RaisingDoctors.com.

REFERENCE LETTERS

When it comes to reference letters, which are required as part of the application, the primary consideration is picking referees who will only speak highly about your child, although some medical schools may request reference letters from physicians or professors in specific disciplines.

If there is a good chance the referee would be reluctant or might say anything truly negative, then your child should not ask that individual for a reference letter. If a referee says something negative about an applicant, it doesn't go unnoticed.

Another factor to consider is whether referees can write well. For my own application I only picked people who I already knew could write effectively.

I also picked people who I trusted to complete and submit the references on time. One late reference letter can make your child ineligible for the application cycle they have applied for.

As mentioned in Chapter 2, some medical schools may request reference letters from an applicant's premedical committee if they have recently graduated from a postsecondary institution.

PREPARING FOR INTERVIEW DAY

Before my interview I listened to a podcast provided by the admissions office at the medical school where I had applied in which two medical students shared how they had prepared for their own interviews.

One had looked up common interview questions and practiced with two different people. Another had hung up a motivational yoga poster and used it for inspiration in the weeks and days leading up to the interview.

There are many ways that applicants can prepare for interviews. The types of questions and interview formats vary and differ from school to school and may also change over time.

This is how my medical school interview day went, but your child may have a very different interview experience:

I was as tired as any mom with young children. My daughter was still waking up at night, but I had to stay focused on the interview for just one day.

I arrived early, wearing a brand-new pair of dress shoes, a professional-looking dress, nylons, and my most formal suit jacket.

I saw other applicants, most of whom were also wearing dark suits, milling around the waiting area and making small talk, but I waited by myself on a bench until the interviews began.

First up was a group interview. We took turns talking and discussing the scenario we were given. No one dominated the group. Everyone gave space for others to contribute what they wanted to say.

I remember how polished some people's answers seemed to me and I felt old compared to everyone in the group. Then, before I knew it, it was over.

In between interviews, I overheard some of the applicants talking about where else they had gotten interviews, about flying to and from them, or having to fly to the same city twice because the different medical schools there had their interviews a few weeks apart.

I had my individual interviews and multiple mini interviews. I remember having to take a step back while answering one of the questions and admitting that I would probably be at a loss for what to do in the given situation. I remember not understanding one of the questions at all and fumbling my way through as I drew on a piece of paper. When the bell rang for the last multiple mini interview, I stood, ready to go on to the next one, but there weren't any more. It was all over!

All the applicants went and sat in a room for a brief presentation. I overheard a woman sitting in front of me saying, "Oh, I liked that question."

I started to get a headache. I was probably dehydrated from still breastfeeding, not drinking enough water, and being in a high-pres-

sure, high-stress situation all day. By the end of the presentation, my head was pounding. I left exhausted, but it was over. I had done it and the decision was now out of my hands.

DOTTING I'S AND CROSSING T'S

Meeting deadlines is extremely important in the application process.

No matter what, your child must make sure to send in a complete, error-free application either early (if the school accepts students on a rolling basis) or on time. Transcripts, MCAT scores, reference letters, and other deliverables must all be submitted in a timely manner to even be considered.

Remember, for all interviews, your child should be professionally dressed in formal business attire whenever possible, be neatly groomed, and treat everyone respectfully. They should make their best possible effort to converse with others in ways that are socially appropriate and make a good first impression.

After the interview, it may be appropriate for your child to follow up with a thank you card to emphasize continued interest in being selected. They should also send thank you cards to referees to show appreciation for reference letters as well as anyone who helped with interview practice or any other aspects of the application process. People appreciate being thanked for their time and advice.

It goes without saying that all interactions with the admissions office, whether accepted, declined, or waitlisted, should be courteous and respectful.

If applicants are not accepted into medical school, they may wish to apply again the following year, or at a later time. With this in mind, it's important for your child to maintain relationships with referees and anyone else who helped or could yet help with the process of applying to medical school.

CHAPTER 6:

HOW YOU CAN HELP AS A PARENT

Now that you have a general understanding of medical school admissions, let's look at how you as a parent can help your child succeed at applying to medical school.

WHAT TO KEEP AND DOCUMENT

Even if your child is very young, start a binder, a file folder, or a file box to keep track of activities, experiences, and accomplishments.

For things like progress cards and certificates, a binder may suffice. You can buy clear pockets to avoid punching holes in your child's important papers. You may need a box for larger, irregularly shaped objects.

Even if not all items are relevant for a medical school application, you can still keep them to jog your child's memory when the time comes to apply and write about life experiences and successes. You can even keep school assignments or arts and crafts. You can take photos of larger items to store electronically.

One day my mother brought me a large file box of all my old stuff from school including book reports, research projects, poetry and stories that I had written, drawings, yearbooks, certificates, medals, and trophies.

This was one of the reasons I was able to write about my high school student council experience; my high school yearbook contained a summary of what my team had accomplished.

By the time I applied to medical school, however, most of the work I did when I was a child was no longer relevant. I no longer needed copies of my junior high newspaper for which I was the editor, nor the many colorful certificates with star stickers that my second grade teacher had given me for doing my homework. But, if I had been a younger applicant, I might have talked more about my activities from high school. The point is, save *everything* because it might be enormously helpful for a successful application.

LEGITIMACY AND VERIFIABILITY MATTER

Applying to medical school, I learned what types of activities, accomplishments, and qualifications were valued and what weren't.

For example, medical schools may restrict the types of publications that applicants list on their application to only include certain categories of publications that are well respected by the profession.

That said, it takes practice and experience to do research and write articles that academic journals will publish. Submitting written work to be published through a variety of channels (newspapers, blogs, anthologies, etc.) can help your child develop the skills needed to write well and have their work accepted for established publications.

Note that medical schools may require roles/jobs, experiences, and other achievements or activities to be **verifiable**, meaning that there must be a person or an organization who can confirm your child's involvement or the work they did. For example, I had a Bronze Cross from the Life Saving Society of Canada; there is a database of all award-holders on the internet that anyone can access to verify this.

As another example, established institutions such as The Royal Conservatory can confirm whether an applicant has achieved a certain level of education in their music training.

If your child attains a high level of mastery in any skill, the organization that oversees their training should be able to verify their achievement, but you may want to check to be sure. Many smaller businesses, for example, do not have a database that keeps track of individuals' accomplishments. If your child trains for only a short period of time, if there is high staff turnover at the organization, or if your child cannot locate the people whom they worked with after many years, there may not be anyone who can verify their participation.

For that reason, for the purposes of a medical school application, it's better to stick with certain activities and organizations for a long time and continue to advance in a few areas, rather than dabble in many different hobbies or interests that cannot be verified.

I have undertaken several unsupervised projects, but always ensure that I find legitimate ways to present or prove my work. I submit abstracts to present original work as posters or presentations at conferences or find organizations to partner with who can verify my projects. I have even had some projects featured in the media, which I have been able to cite as proof of my work.

One example that I could not include in my own medical school application was a certificate of bilingualism that I received from my school board at the end of high school for having completed the French immersion program. When I contacted the school board, they had no database or record of who had received this certificate. After 13 years in the French immersion program, the only thing that I could include in my application related to my training in French was one university-level French course, which appeared on my transcripts.

For titled roles or jobs, your child should maintain an up-to-date curriculum vitae (CV). It's also important to have a separate file or notebook that includes the following basic information:

- Position start and end dates
- Hours worked
- Name, location, and contact information of organization
- Name and contact information of immediate supervisor
- Job description

It's a good idea for your child to write a short memo about the role or job, including what they learned, what they would have changed, and the ways in which they found the experience impactful. This will help them remember the experience more clearly, even years later.

One of the small businesses I worked for 20 years ago no longer existed by the time I applied for medical school. All I had was the name of my supervisor. Fortunately, I was able to track the individual down on social media. They still remembered me!

Long before I applied for medical school, I had donated all my medals and trophies to a charity to be recycled. I kicked myself when I realized I no longer had proof that I had received a specific award because I had given it away. Unfortunately, the school didn't keep records of who had won that award!

Luckily, I had an old photo in an album that showed one of my teachers presenting me with the award. I scanned the photo, looked up the teacher on the internet, and emailed them the photo asking them whether they would verify the award for me.

With this in mind, I recommend taking photos whenever your child receives an award. It also makes sense to write down the name of the teacher who presented it.

Once capable enough to maintain and update a CV, your child should continue to document:

- Research or science activities

- Original published work (prose, poetry, articles, academic papers, books)
- Dates, locations, and titles of presentations
- Certificates, medals, trophies, or other awards
- Evidence of grants or scholarships
- Media appearances or features (e.g., in blogs, magazines, newspapers, podcasts, or videos)

Managing collegial relationships with potential verifiers is essential to the process of applying to medical school. If your child is having trouble getting something verified or getting a reference on time, encourage respectful persistence in any query.

If a referee is not replying or cooperating, then it may be time to ask someone else to write that reference. In my case, a payroll employee would not reply with the information I requested. I eventually had to seek out and talk to this person's supervisor to be assured that they could verify my employment with them.

SPEND TIME WITH DOCTORS

In medical school, a large proportion of medical students have a family member who is a physician, whether a parent, sibling, spouse, or a more distant relative.

On one side of my family are both doctors and pharmacists. Although many of my relatives have passed on, I found myself spending more time with doctors on my husband's side of the family after I got married. One of my best friends is also a doctor. Although I never specifically intended to befriend doctors, as it has turned out, I now enjoy the company of many.

For the purpose of applying to medical school, spending time with doctors can come with many advantages.

RECOGNIZE THAT DOCTORS ARE PEOPLE TOO

When you are surrounded by doctors, the idea of *being* a doctor becomes very normal.

From spending time with doctors, your child will come to see that doctors are normal human beings. They are not perfect, and they have their faults. They do normal things like playing sports or video games, doing housework, cooking, shopping, and spending time with their families.

Getting to know doctors may also help your child see that "ordinary" people can become doctors if they work hard; they can gain an understanding of the reality of being a doctor; and see first-hand how a medical career progresses. Your child may be able to ask questions and get an inside look at the profession in terms of job satisfaction, work-life balance, and the financial side.

GAIN COMFORT WITH WHAT DOCTORS DO

Many medical students whose parents are doctors seem more comfortable doing the job of doctors. Over their lives they have watched their parents administer first aid and care for family members, or might have learned some medicine from them.

Not everyone is cut out to take care of people who are sick or deal with medical emergencies. But having a doctor-figure present earlier in life can help young people learn about what doctors do on a day-to-day basis.

After only a year of medical school, I found myself more at ease explaining the human body to my son, and answering questions like, "Where does pee come from?" I practiced physical exams on my kids, and after going over the exam routines and maneuvers dozens of times, my son would start to prompt and remind me of things that I forgot to say.

Pretty soon, my daughter, who was two at the time, would instruct me to sit on the couch so she could examine me, toy stethoscope around her neck. She would say, "I'm going to be a doctor. I'm going to take care of people."

Kids are impressionable. Having positive role models and experiences related to the medical profession early on can prime them for a career as a doctor.

UNDERSTAND PROFESSIONAL EXPECTATIONS

Doctors understand the culture of medicine. They know that medical schools have, historically, mainly accepted applicants who are academically high achieving, "professional," and squeaky clean.

Anyone with one too many skeletons in their closet, or who has been involved in embarrassing incidents witnessed by the public or posted online, may have these issues come back to haunt them if they pursue medicine as a career. This is a bit of a conundrum because doctors must sometimes take risks, go out on a limb, or stick their necks out to advocate for their patients and even for themselves. The culture of medicine is slowly changing, however, as more people with diverse competencies and lived experiences join the profession.

Many doctors have also been on committees that review medical school applications and interview applicants. They may have sound, up-to-date advice for applying to medical school, especially if their experiences of screening applicants reflect the practices and values of the school where your child is applying.

In short, building relationships with doctors may help your child to understand what is expected of medical school applicants and physicians well in advance, and help them to become the ideal applicant.

KNOW HOW TO PREPARE FOR
MEDICAL TRAINING

Doctors know what must be learned in medical training. They can better ensure their children are prepared for the material presented in medical school, including subjects like cellular biology, human physiology, anatomy, and emergency medicine. Even skills like administering procedures, performing physical exams, or examining specimens can become second nature for a student who has a parent or family member who can teach them these practices.

Some parents with experience in medicine or academia may get their children involved in research activities from a young age or encourage their children to seek out such opportunities.

If you are not a medical professional yourself, it may be difficult to give your child this kind of advantage. That said, bear in mind that preexisting knowledge and experience in these domains is not necessarily a prerequisite at many medical schools. Your child can seek out relevant knowledge and research or clinical experiences when it makes sense for them, and when they are more able to do so.

In medical school, most students will have an advantage in some areas, but not in others. The world of medicine is vast, and no one can know it all. Be reassured: the subject matter your child finds the most interesting is the right domain for them to study.

Naturally, not all applicants who have physicians as parents get into medical school. Many applicants with perfect GPAs who have studied all the relevant subjects and done all the "right" things still do not get into medical school.

Today's medical school applicant must not only know what medical schools require, but also have insight into who they are as a person, and what made them that way.

No number of physician family members or friends can tell your child who they are and what their most defining life experiences are. They must figure it out on their own, and then communicate it as best as they can in their application.

CHAPTER 7:

PARENTING VALUES AND PRIORITIES

Parents often wonder how much emphasis to place on various priorities, from education to extracurricular activities, and the nurturing of various values, beliefs, and attitudes. These are important considerations no matter what career your child may wish to pursue.

PURSUE PASSIONS, PURPOSE, AND STRENGTHS

Special interests, hobbies, and projects provide alternative outlets and balance for children and older students—something we all need. Most healthy children and adults need an assortment of activities to maintain a balanced lifestyle.

My kids learned to bike, swim, and skate so they can enjoy more diverse activities with their friends and our family as they get older. But beyond a basic skill level, I don't feel they need to spend a great deal of time or energy on these activities unless they truly enjoy them and are self-motivated to work at them.

As adults, we often have things we would have liked to learn or would like to spend time learning now. No matter how many activities we sign our children up for, and how far they go, there will always be another activity they would have wanted to do or another new hobby to consider.

Many people have lamented to me that they didn't put enough time into playing the piano when they were young. They are surprised to hear that I feel I should have quit playing the piano sooner. I wasn't one of those kids who lived and breathed music. I didn't create or compose my own original pieces. I had no natural talent in it, nor the obsessive drive to truly become masterful at it.

Although playing the piano may have come with some benefits, I believe that spending so much time and effort on something your child doesn't absolutely love is increasingly a mistake.

If your child doesn't show a real interest in something, let them decide whether they want to come back to it as an adult. Sometimes it's a blessing to give up activities so that true passions and strengths have a chance to emerge.

When deciding on pursuits with your child, ask yourself these questions:

- Do they derive joy from it or are they passionate about it?
- Do they get a sense of purpose or meaning from it?
- Would they eventually be able to perform on the world stage at it?

Whether your child intends to include a particular activity on their medical school application in the future or not, they are more likely to succeed at it if they love doing it and are good at it.

For the next generation of children, being a big fish in a small pond at anything will not be enough to make a living. *We live in an increasingly global, digital, and competitive economy.* According to Seth Godin, author of *The Dip*, it pays a disproportionate premium to be the very best at something. People flock to whatever or whoever is "number one," and are willing to pay much more for best-in-class than for their competitors.[22]

"Number two" only gets market share by doing something uniquely different or charging so much less that people are willing to compromise on what they truly would have wanted if it weren't for the price.

Would you want your operation performed by the best surgeon or the second-best surgeon for the job? Most likely, you would want the very best surgeon you could find.

That's why, in this global economy, it increasingly only pays to be the best in your field at something.

This also applies to being a best-in-class generalist. For example, in the medical field, general practitioners and diagnosticians need to have a broad knowledge that they can draw upon to help their patients. A handyman may also be a generalist who has a variety of tools and skills to fix different kinds of household problems. Best-in-class generalists get the best and most customers and work opportunities compared to other generalists.

It's possible your child has a very specific interest or skill. Should you support them even if their passion has nothing to do with a career plan or if it might not be possible to make a living from it? It depends.

We all need to do things we enjoy, but when it comes to hobbies, it's also valuable to pick activities that we can cultivate and improve on. This concept ties into the Sparketype discussion in Chapter 4.[23]

With an activity that your child enjoys in mind, consider these questions:

- Does your child learn from, produce, solve, or improve anything from the activity?
- Do they perform in front of, lead, teach, advocate for, advise, or nurture others?

If the answer is "Yes," this activity may help your child to develop and gain skills in their preferred type of work. Excelling at something demonstrates that your child has the discipline to develop mastery, which is applicable to careers in medicine.

Going further, taking on a formal role or participating in the activity at a competitive or professional level would make such an experience verifiable and could contribute to a successful medical school application.

Although, there are no established or recognized markets for many hobbies or interests, some people can still find ways to capitalize on their passions and make money from them. If they love the work so much, they would do it anyway and either be recognized for it—regardless of the income potential—or keep doing it simply for pleasure and as a break from other forms of work.

LATENT GIFTS

I didn't really discover the work I was meant to do until my thirties: My work involves engaging in broad-based learning that connects the dots between different ideas and gives me new insights into the domains I'm interested in. Much of my extracurricular work in and out of medicine are applications of this, including this book.

I'm not sure if I would have had the cognitive ability to do this type of work when I was younger, but I derive a great deal of meaning, purpose, and satisfaction from it... now that I'm older. I create things that I am uniquely able to produce. I have even become more spiritual since arriving at this type of work, because I feel that I understand my place in the universe and how I am connected to it.

If I had developed these abilities at a younger age, I might have accomplished more to date, but I also believe that everything happens for a reason. The work I do now could not have been done as efficiently or as enjoyably without the internet. The World Wide Web and social media have greatly facilitated the learning and sharing of information and ideas. I discovered the work that was right for me when it presented itself and I was in a position to accept it.

The funny thing is that to prepare for this type of "learning" work, I needed outstanding reading skills. Obsessively reading dozens of novels every month as a child actually prepared me for what I was meant to do in my life. But to my parents, teachers, and classmates at the time, I must have just looked like an extraordinary bookworm.

You may have a child who watches a lot of TV, plays video games, or surfs the Web all day. The line between frivolous fun, serious work, and unhealthy patterns of behavior may be blurry at times. In a world where screen time may be hazardous to both adults and children, but where eSports, app-building, and working at a computer all day have become normal, it is not always clear what to do as a parent. You are, however, responsible for the decisions you make with respect to your child's use of technology.

As the parent, you need to gauge whether your child has a healthy productive interest or if there is an underlying problem. If you have a health concern about your child, seek professional advice, but also consider the possibility that your child's hobby could be a gift.

ALL EXPERIENCES MATTER

Your strengths can become your child's too if you are able to teach them and they are willing to learn from you. If you currently practice a trade or work at a skilled job, teach them what you can.

If your native tongue is not English, it's best to teach it to your child early, if you plan to teach it at all. My husband has been teaching our kids his native Chinese language, Teochew, since they were born, for example.

If you're a good cook, teach your child to cook as though they might open a restaurant one day. If you're a master weaver, teach them your art, including every fancy knot and stitch you know. There may not be much of a market for homemade items when corporate giants are able to mass manufacture thousands of products every day, but your child will still gain unique skills and attributes from practicing an artistic endeavor that results in a finished product to show for their efforts. They may successfully produce or invent other useful things one day by adapting the skills they learned from you.

None of these skills will necessarily go to waste even if your child is pursuing medicine. The medical profession and healthcare in general need people with unique and special skills and perspectives to bring novel ideas to old problems, and to apply age-old practices to new problems.

There is no reason that the knowledge and skills your child gains in a completely different discipline or trade cannot be applied to medicine to better human life in some way.

Although I can't say that becoming a YouTube star is the way to get into medical school, there are undoubtedly skills to be gained from hobbies like this. It takes practice and discipline to excel in a competitive environment and perform or improvise, on stage or on video, in front of a large audience. Likewise, it takes practice and discipline to learn scripts, maneuvers, and procedures to perform physical exams or even operate on patients.

Medical trainees and professionals need strong presentation skills to pass tests of their physical exam skills as well as over the course of their careers. So don't discount endeavors in the performing arts or professional sports, which essentially require competitors to *perform*.

Right now, I appear to have one child who is athletic and nurturing and one who likes to build/make things and perform in front of others. Although my kids are still young and their interests or strengths may change, I plan to give them more exposure to opportunities that cater to their strengths and interests as they grow up. If I have the means to support them in developing these areas, even a little bit, how could I not?

PROVIDE AUTONOMY FOR ALL THE RIGHT REASONS

I sometimes see videos on social media of small children who are cooking and feeding themselves. Meanwhile, when my kids were the same age, I was still dressing and feeding them breakfast in a frenzy every morning to get them out the door for school and daycare. It's not always fair to compare between households, but it's easy to recognize that children have varying levels of agency and autonomy, depending on their situations or that of their parents.

CULTIVATE AN ATTITUDE OF SERVICE

Despite our hectic North American routines, it's still important to give children responsibilities and autonomy. Those who do things themselves learn and appreciate what it means to be independent and self-sufficient.

One way to do this is to give your child chores. If they are not cooking, they can at least set the table or clean up after meals. Get them to help with laundry or do their own when they're able. Let them pack their school bag and remember to do their own homework. If they forget their library book once, they will remember the next time. If they leave their snack or wallet at home, they may go hungry for a meal, but they will make sure to bring it the following day. Let them score the grades they are going to score without your help. This will allow you to see where their true strengths and interests lie.

I have met people who did extremely well in school and even won scholarships because of their helicopter parents. These were the parents who took their children to the library every week, helped them to pick out books for school projects, or did some of the research themselves, and corrected the homework before allowing them to hand it in.

Other parents, while not over-helping with homework, reason that as long as their child is doing well in school and staying out of trouble, they can do whatever they want with the rest of their time.

The trouble arises when children learn that everyone else exists to serve *them* by cooking, cleaning, caring, and even doing their work for them.

Some children learn to under-value the work and contributions of others and end up putting their own needs above the needs of others. We only have to watch a few episodes of Dr. Phil to see how doing too much for our children can cause some extreme and serious issues in young adults, like obsessing over becoming Instagram famous or staying in bed for months at a time.

Whatever your parenting style or beliefs, it's important to frame any work, responsibilities, autonomy, and even independence in terms of service to a greater cause, a common good, or service to others. Whether this is done in the context of religion or spirituality, or as service to community or humankind, cultivating an attitude of service is necessary for all contributing members of society, and especially for a profession like medicine.

Medical students and doctors must serve others. They serve their patients, their institutions, their team members, and all humanity. For people who have faith, they may serve God.

If you or your child view their day-to-day purpose as "learning" or "doing well in school," make sure they know *why* that's their purpose. It is not so they can grow up to be better, wealthier, or more successful than everyone else, or only to bring honor, respect, or abundance to you or your family. **There is always a greater purpose at stake, for each person, for doctors and people who want to be doctors, and for their families—even if it is to simply survive.**

FOSTER RESPECT AND APPRECIATION FOR ESSENTIAL WORK

If our children's schoolwork, premedical or medical studies, or their work as a doctor is so important, serves others, or even saves lives...should they be doing "menial" tasks like housework at all?

The truth is, it's a privilege to do important work that changes lives and changes the world. Most people would want to do significant, meaningful work that they feel well aligned with if they could. It is inherently rewarding to do it. But not everyone has the ability or the opportunity to do desirable work. And essential work must still be done.

In October 2019, a member of Congress in the United States, Katie Porter, asked Mark Zuckerberg if he would do the job of a Facebook content moderator, reviewing the darkest, most violent and heinous material on the social media platform, for even an hour. The work of content moderators is difficult and even traumatizing.

Zuckerberg responded by stating he was "not sure that it would best serve our community for me to spend that much time" on such a task,[24] despite the fact that he would not make any less money than usual for spending one hour as a content moderator.

But what if it *would* best serve "our community" for Zuckerberg to spend time doing this undesirable work? He may in fact already spend the odd hour reviewing content on Facebook. The reason why this much-needed work is not more highly valued and not better compensated is only because our societal and economic structures do not reflect our societal and human values.

There may be tasks that trainees and clinicians find to be undesirable, *but they still have to do them* as it stands right now. The work that one doesn't want to do, but that still has to be done is valuable. Learning this early may help your child to have realistic expectations as they grow older and respect the work of colleagues, co-workers, staff, and medical learners, just as we should appreciate the difficult, stressful, and time-consuming yet important work of physicians.

No one is actually above doing any kind of work, unless we have a solution for this work that makes it possible for no one to have to do it at all.

HOUSEWORK IS HEALTHY

Another way to look at some forms of work is as a break from other work. Even billionaires need time to decompress and downtime doing the mundane. Sometimes that's when the best ideas strike.

In 2019, Melinda Gates published a new book resulting in widespread interest in the fact that the Gates' wash their dishes together every night as a practice that maintains an equal and balanced partnership and a strong marriage.[25]

How is it that the simple, boring, everyday task of washing dishes can generate so much media attention? Apparently, we collectively believe that rich, famous, "important" people don't do, or shouldn't do housework. But it turns out that they do, and for them it can be beneficial and not just a chore.

While I was in my first year of medical school, I did as little housework as possible. I tried to spend almost all my time on the highest yield activities: studying, homework, and spending time with my kids. I wouldn't allow myself to spend time doing something that allowed my mind to just rest, wander, or do nothing.

Because of this, I was always on edge. Not only that, but I was performing suboptimally because my brain wasn't getting enough rest between study sessions, and I felt like I was studying *all the time.*

I can now appreciate doing *more* housework and mundane tasks like grocery shopping. These chores serve the very important purpose of helping me maintain a healthy balance.

RAISE A SELF-SUFFICIENT ADULT

The amount of housework your child is responsible for is something that you need to continually reevaluate. Although having your child do some chores is both healthy and helpful, too many may hinder their chances of getting into medical school by taking time away from their schoolwork. Remember that the average GPA for gaining admission to certain medical schools is trending towards 4.0.

Some students have parents who help them regularly with schoolwork. While one student spends an hour on a school project, another student and parent may together spend 10 hours on the same assignment.

Although not fair, it is a reality that needs to be contended with. Intensive parenting may give children an advantage to some extent, by helping them to outperform their peers at an early age.

In his book *David and Goliath*, Malcolm Gladwell demonstrates that people who gain confidence early on in less competitive academic environments can become more successful over the course of their lives than people who struggled in more competitive settings.[26]

In terms of academics, children who score higher grades eventually get more recognition in terms of accolades, such as awards, grants, or scholarships. And there may be a legacy effect. After receiving a verifiable award, a student could be better positioned to receive other awards or funding and to impress admissions committees of medical schools.

Children whose parents don't have the time, skills, or other resources to help them get good grades are unfortunately at a disadvantage in this respect. This is not right, and it is something that must continue to be addressed and overcome, with changes to structures that currently perpetuate systemic inequity.

Conversely, autonomously motivated students may thrive despite, or even *because of*, having less parental help. They succeed because they have agency, they care about doing well, and they don't need to be reminded or cajoled into doing their homework. They may even enjoy doing the work.

Fostering autonomy and a sense of agency in your child, therefore, is vitally important.

If you can achieve a balance between supporting and helping your child with what is needed from an adult, and giving them an appropriate amount of autonomy for their stage of development and level of competence, they may gain more confidence because of what they personally accomplish.

In other words, parents need to allow their children to fall and fail sometimes in order for them to step up and realize what they are capable of doing. Other times, children take responsibility because it is the parent who falls or fails. For example, when I misplaced my wallet, my son remembered where it was. After receiving praise, each time we went out, he would remind me to bring my wallet. It gave him a sense of pride to do something helpful and important, and allowed him to practice taking some responsibility.

Family units are organic, in a sense. You may have someone in your family who always holds it together, someone who is less predictable, someone who is generally successful, someone who is more laid-back, someone who gives, and someone who is better at receiving. But these are not necessarily fixed roles specific to each person.

If one person steps out of character or changes roles, the others will tend to adapt and rearrange their roles for the family to survive as a unit. If you feel that you or someone else is doing too much or too little, if possible, you may wish to try taking on a different role for a change and see what happens.

At the end of the day, you cannot become a doctor for your child. You cannot do their work of treating patients, taking licensing exams, practicing physical exams, taking the MCAT, or writing medical school applications, even if you want to.

Students must put the work in themselves if they really want to become a medical professional. Your role may be to get out of their way and give them space to follow their interests.

Medicine is a long and hard road. There is no sense in your child pursuing it unless they want it for themselves, have a sense of agency to do the work of applying to medical school, and have years of personal experience scoring well on exams and schoolwork they did on their own.

Even then, they may at times need to live at home or move back home for you to take care of them, just to cope with the heavy demands of medical training.

One of the best things you can do for a child interested in medicine is to give them the autonomy they need to function independently at a high level as a self-sufficient adult. This will serve them no matter what path they pursue.

CHAPTER 8:

DOING THE SELF WORK

The principle of working on yourself first (rather than working on your child), is an important one in any discussion where relationships are involved. If you work on yourself, your child will invariably benefit, especially since self-awareness is a valuable asset for a medical school applicant.

RAISE YOUR OWN SELF-AWARENESS

To some extent, children's ability to gain self-awareness and insight is limited by whether or not the people closest to them are able to do so. Working on your own self-awareness is one way to help your child develop insight. When one person (in a family, for example) starts to operate from a place grounded in truth, this has a ripple effect on the people around that person.

If you currently have unresolved problems or issues from the past, deal with them to the best of your ability. Get professional help if necessary.

- Start prioritizing your health or self-care if you have not been doing so.

- Simplify your life if you're drowning in clutter or complexity.

- Establish boundaries with people who do not treat you fairly.

- Consider the possibility of healing from whatever is hurting you.
- Allow your beliefs to be challenged.

Whatever the situation, do not be complacent. You can only be effective at helping your child be their best—whether applying to medical school or in any aspect of life—if you are talking the talk and walking the walk yourself.

You may know from experience that it is difficult to maintain a relationship or even a conversation with someone exhibiting poor self-awareness—even if it's a family member. While as a parent you may be frustrated with your child over certain things, your child may be equally frustrated with you if you cannot meet them where they are.

But you can try to become more self-aware, which will enable you to communicate and relate effectively with your child. I'm not suggesting you compete with them or try to always be right, but rather, to work on engendering self-awareness in yourself and in your relationship with them.

Most likely, up to this point, you have done the best you could with what you have. But by reading this book, you may have some new ideas on how to do things differently. For the sake of your child, always work on yourself first, instead of "working on" or trying to change your child.

You cannot change another person, only yourself.

IDENTIFY PROBLEM AREAS

Here's a list of questions to help you identify areas that you can address in your own life, and that are helpful for the parent of someone who may want to apply to medical school.

1. When a family member brings you bad news, do you explode in anger or express disapproval? How can you better respond to risks, mistakes, setbacks, or failures?

2. Do you feel unsafe at home? Do you ever fear for anyone's safety or is anyone worried about you? Are you unable to talk to anyone outside of your own house on a regular and frequent basis? If so, who can you ask for help?

3. Do you talk about people in a negative way in front of your child? Do you complain about doctors or the medical establishment? If so, what is the issue that really needs to be addressed?

4. Do you condemn, disrespect, lash out, or curse at people at work, in public, or on social media? How can you communicate more respectfully with others?

5. Do you feel you maintain appropriate boundaries with others at home and at work? If not, how can you take action to prioritize your needs appropriately and set much-needed boundaries?

6. Do you punish others with the silent treatment to teach them a lesson or "ghost" them to avoid talking about a difficult topic? How can you manage your relationships in more loving and assertive ways?

7. Do you praise things or people you believe are better or more righteous than others and put them on a pedestal? What do you idolize? What would it look like for you to prioritize equality and inclusion or help those who are disadvantaged?

8. Is there anything you deeply regret about your life? Or are you honestly living your best possible life?

9. Do you, at some level, feel you are not good enough, or not worthy? Are you lonely? What if you can still achieve your own goals, dreams, or ambitions . . . or find your own people?

10. Is there any aspect of your own work, home, or parenting situation that frustrates you? What small change can you make to improve your situation?

11. Would you support your child or another family member to see a professional or an advisor of their own choosing (e.g., physician, social worker, mental health professional, teacher, religious leader, life coach, etc.)? What if your child was already a medical student and needed professional support?

12. Would you consider seeking professional help for yourself?

This is not an exhaustive list, but it may help you consider what you can do as a parent—to benefit your child and yourself.

Many of the questions on the list deal with personal safety issues. We all have a basic need for safety that must be met before we can achieve higher goals. If you, your child, or anyone else in your household does not feel safe in some way, this will be having a profound effect on your child's ability to fully thrive.

The latter part of the list addresses limiting beliefs and tendencies that may be affecting your big life decisions and everyday choices. If you consider these questions and realize you are not being or doing what you want, tread carefully. Incredible turmoil and stress can come from trying to change too much at a time.

I've known people who took massive action to better their lives: moved from one city or even country to another, quit jobs to start new careers, separated from partners, or sold everything they owned. Although these decisions may work for some people, especially the small percentage of people whose good news stories you may read about, I do not advise taking drastic measures without some sort of safety net, nor do I recommend doing too much at once.

Unless your safety is at risk, it is a much more sustainable approach to make small or incremental changes from where you are and to try to make things work with what you have. If you are unhappy with your job, your boss, or your workplace, for example, before you call it quits, try to make small changes that will better align your work with your preferences and needs.

Before having my kids, for example, I worked for a company as a business analyst where I switched jobs seven times in seven years. I moved departments, changed bosses, and tried different projects. There were many times when I truly appreciated my work and colleagues. But eventually I did not feel it was a fit for the long term and so I left the company.

Sometimes it is necessary to step in and make changes. When one of my kids was hitting me, I knew I could not let that behavior continue, especially as someone with a serious interest in preventing violence. I learned to fairly enforce consequences and, in this case, eventually took my child's toy away. *It worked* and I am all for doing what works when it comes to violence.

Working through the unique issues that may come up for you may help your child to not only apply to medical school, but also keep unhealthy tendencies in check or be better prepared for life in general.

DO WHAT IS RIGHT FOR YOU

Although this is a book for parents, and I believe I'm at least as good as any other parent, I am also *no better* than other parents. As parents, we all struggle with some things and we all make mistakes.

You do not necessarily need to change anything to improve the chances of your child getting into medical school or otherwise becoming successful in life. It is up to you to decide whether my self-examining questions are relevant to you, or to prioritize any issues that arise from your own self-exploration and self-awareness. Most importantly, do what is right for you.

Interestingly, as I gained more awareness about myself and my relationships, everyone close to me also became more self-aware in parallel. At one point, for example, I realized that I could refuse to act as an intermediary between certain family members. These family members, who weren't talking to one another, eventually had to take responsibility for the problem themselves once they understood that I would no longer serve as a workaround. Our boundaries have shifted slightly, and I feel more mutual respect and acceptance from those around me.

The point is that increasing your own self-awareness may help you, your child, or even others in your life, whether a successful medical school application or other goals are the end result.

Whatever comes up for you in this section, give yourself credit. You are a good parent. No matter your child's age, you have made it this far just by being you and doing all the things you do!

LOVE FULLY, BE PROUD, AND BE LOUD

I have a parent who seems to be proud of me just for the fact that I exist, even if I don't do anything particularly impressive. In some of my worst moments, this parent gave me unconditional love. From those experiences, I feel I have worth no matter what has happened to me or whatever I have done.

But unfortunately, not everyone has a parent who is proud of them, or feels they were ever seen as good enough. I believe that growing up and living without experiencing unconditional love is a rocky, slippery, and treacherous foundation for self-esteem, self-love, and realizing one's potential.

I have experienced unconditional love. My parents provided me with every opportunity I really needed to succeed in life, and I am extremely grateful for everything they have done for me. Yet I still have moments where I feel I am not enough: I'm not always the best child; I sometimes let them down; or I fail them in some way.

When I gained some awareness of this feeling of "not being enough," I started a practice of visualizing a fictitious moment when my parents were proud of me, *all* of me. I would bask in their love and acceptance for just a few seconds every day, for a few days straight. During those moments, I would allow myself to fully accept their love for me, which was something I had trouble doing, even though they had always given me all the love that I could possibly imagine.

This practice helped to heal the parts in me that felt broken or not fully formed at times and to accept that I had been deserving and worthy of their love all along. It became another spiritual experience I could draw from to fill myself with love when I needed it most.

It is from this place of feeling full of unconditional love that I try to give my kids the love they need to thrive. I am not always successful. Sometimes I don't feel loving at all, and I'm sure my kids can sense those trying moments. But I frequently tell them I love them and that I'm proud of them, for accomplishments and gestures of all sizes, and for no reason at all.

One of my kids sometimes expresses a heartfelt sentiment of gratitude and love when we have special moments as a family. Those are times I treasure and cherish as a parent.

The other started saying, "I'm proud of you, Mom," at just two years old. It feels hard to live up to being the parent of a two-year-old child who tells you how proud they are of you!

REDEFINING THE PROUD PARENT

As a parent, yes, I want to give my kids the means to succeed, but I also want them to be proud to have me as their mom. For me, that means doing the best I can for them so that they can be who they want to be, but I also want the world to be a better place for them to be *in*.

It's not "success" for privileged children to grow smarter, faster, and wealthier than others while performing jobs that serve increasing numbers of people who are jobless, homeless, abandoned, or sick.

If I were to raise doctors, I wouldn't want them to have to shoulder the growing burden of public health crises.

I want each of my kids to know I love them, every part of them, and that I am proud of them. But I want to also love and be proud of myself as a parent, and for me, that means advocating for change where it's needed..

I believe it's important for parents, and perhaps especially parents of doctors, medical trainees, and even medical school applicants, to gain an understanding of public health issues to improve societal problems for the next generation so that the full weight of these problems does not fall on our children. Climate and environment-related issues, lack of access to income and healthcare, poverty and homelessness, discrimination, conflict, extremism, and ableism are just some of the problems that need to be addressed with a sense of urgency.

Our children will be wise to which problems we left unresolved for them to deal with, and which we actually tried to solve. Remember that the task of raising doctors is for the betterment of all. Take action to also raise up many who are being left behind—and be proud.

BE YOUR CHILD'S CHEERLEADER

We all need cheerleaders. In *Cheering for the Children*, Casey Gwinn says, "all children need at least one person to passionately love, cheer for, affirm, encourage, and believe in them."[27]

When my children didn't want to put their faces in the water during swim lessons, I cheered for them, loudly. I cheered for their first glides to the wall. I cheered when they jumped into the pool.

I cheered at skating lessons too, especially when it was difficult for them to get up after a fall.

And then they started reminding me to cheer for them if they tried to do something difficult . . . like walk up a big snowy hill.

I don't always understand what they are trying to accomplish, but I cheer anyway.

Your child needs cheerleaders. Whether they are pursuing a true passion, purpose, or strength, jumping a stepping stone, or simply taking a detour on a more scenic path, they need cheerleaders, and they must find them if they are to do any of these things.

Sometimes they will need you to cheer for them when they choose to defer or quit at something, even if it breaks your heart. Trust that they know what is right for them and who they need cheering for them and when.

Given the importance that our society places on doctors, I believe that my children (like many people) will always view the role of a doctor in a certain venerated light. **It is, therefore, important to be intentional in making it known to them that other pursuits are not lesser, and to mean it.**

You cannot control the narrative that your children will have about you and your role in their endeavors. You can't know if they will thank or blame you for cheering so hard, or not cheering enough. You won't know if they succeeded because you were or you weren't cheering for them, or even though you got in their way, or made things so much more difficult that they had to work extra hard to prove that they wanted something, no matter what.

I cannot tell you to cheer for everything or to cheer all the time, but what I can say is, whether you are cheering (or whether you aren't): *do it (or don't do it) for them—not for you.*

Can you be their cheerleader? Yes, you can.

CHAPTER 9:

UNDERSTANDING MEDICAL STUDENT STRESS

It was my first year in medical school and I needed help.

I needed rest, care, and time.

I felt the same way as I did after my first baby, the same way that many mothers feel after having a baby—like I needed to go back to the hospital and have other people take care of me.

If only I could just not wake up at all, then I wouldn't have to deal with any of this.

No. I didn't want to "not wake up."

I just wanted to retire and lie on a beach in the Caribbean for the rest of my life.

No. What I actually wanted, what I actually NEEDED was a vacation, even if it was just a staycation. Two weeks straight of lying in bed.

But I was only in Course 1, the very first major course in medical school. How could I explain to anyone that I already needed a break?

- *Because I had a one-year-old who refused to sleep before midnight every night.*

- *Because I hadn't slept for more than six hours a night for months.*
- *Because I was experiencing postpartum stress, a normal and common (but misunderstood) issue that many parents experience.*
- *Because I felt like my kids were being torn out of my arms and I missed them terribly.*
- *Because I wasn't yet identifying as a "medical student," but I had to keep up with doing everything that a medical student does.*
- *Because I was having an identity crisis.*
- *Because I regretted not making a request to defer medical school for another year, and now it might be too late.*
- *Because I had yet to embrace the likelihood that the best time for me to be in medical school was right then, at that particular moment, as a mother in her late thirties, no earlier, no later.*

I felt like I was on a slippery slope. If I didn't finish Course 1, I might not finish medical school. And I had to finish medical school.

What would I tell my kids? That it was too hard? That I quit because it was hard?

No, I could not stop.

And that is how I survived my first year of medical school.

When I first started medical school, I revisited this dialog in my head almost every day for weeks, perhaps even months. It was one of the most painful times of my life, because of the combination of stressors I was experiencing.

Starting medical school is one of the biggest changes that a person can go through in life.

Think of when your first child was born. Chances are that you had to make some serious adjustments to your lifestyle and get used to being a parent. You became responsible for the life of another human being!

While some new parents seem to carry on with their lives like they did before, others experience great difficulty adjusting to a new life with kids—and many have trouble just getting out of the house. Regardless of gender, new parents can experience postpartum stress, anxiety, or depression.

In a similar way, every medical student experiences medical school differently. Some seem to coast through effortlessly, while for others it can be debilitating.

If your child is starting medical school, treat it as one of the biggest transitions they will ever have to make and give them as much support as they need. They are not becoming responsible for just one human's life; they are becoming responsible for the care and health of all human beings. And those are big shoes to fill.

Although my experience is unique to me, many medical students have felt some of the pain I described in one way or another.

To read more first-person stories of medical trainees, visit the following websites:

Canada: perspectivesinmedicine.ca

United States: in-training.org

PREMEDICAL PROBLEMS

For many students, problems with stress begin well before starting medical school.

Many parents of straight-A students routinely ask where the other 2 percent went if their children come home with a score of 98 percent on an exam. Competitive students learn to appeal grades and fight tooth and nail for every last percentage point, because nothing short of a perfect score is good enough.

For some students, this situation is already untenable. In fact, Kaplan surveyed 400 premeds and reported in 2020 that 37 percent seriously contemplated abandoning their medical career plans because of the amount of stress involved.[28]

The report stated that students may feel trapped in their career plans and a cycle of constantly comparing themselves with competitive peers. Fifty-seven percent of respondents said that alcohol and other drug use is common among premedical peers experiencing stress.[29]

Unfortunately, these issues may be exacerbated in medical training, or as I've been problematically told, "it will only get worse." Right now, anyone pursuing medicine as a career must withstand significant stress and have a high tolerance for uncertainty.

WORKLOADS AND SCHEDULES

Medical students often say that being in medical school is like "drinking from a firehose." They are inundated with information about injuries, emergencies, and diseases, and although they do not have to remember every detail, they need to know enough to potentially identify and treat the many various medical conditions and clinical presentations they will encounter.

Medical students have mandatory lectures, group sessions, and clinical experiences—and little control over their schedules. Being a medical student is basically like having a full-time job with most of the time already scheduled into various activities.

Students must request permission to miss mandatory sessions and usually need to make them up at a later date. This can make it difficult for them to take days off.

In addition to attending 20–30 hours of lectures or sessions per week, most medical students must study every day. They often have deliverables with deadlines to meet, group sessions to prepare for with pre-reading, not to mention also studying for exams.

SINK OR SWIM

For medical students who get behind, there is a massive snow-ball-rolling-down-a-hill effect in terms of the amount of work that accumulates, and it becomes increasingly difficult to catch up. The pace of medical school is hard to describe and can only be fully appreciated by students who have been there. It can feel like a constant sink or swim situation.

Thinking back to the new parent analogy, imagine you neglected to change your baby's diapers for a few days in a row. Your baby would need an emergency intervention! You simply cannot get behind. During the first few months, medical students scramble to adjust to the requirements of their new role and find study methods and resources that work for them.

I remember when the pace started to really accelerate. I sat and cried in my basement for a few minutes before buckling down to stay on top of the material. I wasn't the only one in my class in tears that week.

Many medical students experience serious failures for the first time in their lives because of their workload or other circumstances.

Under these conditions, some students are bound to fail exams or not meet other requirements. This is particularly stressful for students who are accustomed to exceling at school and it can undermine their confidence. Failing exams or other requirements may also set them back, meaning that they have to repeat assignments, tests, courses, or even a year of school.

Finding ways to cope with stress, uncertainty, and the inevitable lack of ability to maintain control and perfection during medical school is incredibly important for medical students.

PERSONAL RELATIONSHIPS

Achieving balance while in medical school can be difficult with respect to relationships with partners, family, and friends. Unfortunately, some students experience relationship and marital breakdowns during medical school.

For students who already have difficulty making time for family, friends, hobbies, interests, or even exercise because of their busy schedules, this can be an especially stressful and isolating experience. Many medical students rely on one another for support, but conversely, they don't want to be stigmatized by classmates for failures they are ashamed of.

These are some of the moments that they may need their parents the most to simply love and support them.

PREPARING FOR THE MATCH

Medical students must undertake career planning over the course of their studies in preparation for matching to a residency program. As part of this they may "shadow" doctors and observe them taking care of patients, attend information sessions, or research different careers and specialties.

Students may also network through clinical and research experiences, or participate in interest groups. They must consistently work towards finding good references and building their portfolios and CVs to compete in the matching process for residency.

Medical students who are effective in their career planning have more positive experiences in medical school because they build a network of physicians interested in supporting them in their careers. Career planning, however, can entail a lot of work, requiring many hours of emails, follow-up, scheduling, and rescheduling.

At first it was difficult for me to find physicians with similar interests to my own, and in my first year of medical school focusing a great deal on career planning would have taken away too much time from my studies and family.

But by the second year, I knew I had to spend more time networking and pursuing my interests if I could. Other students were having more successful clinical experiences because they were working with doctors who had common interests. They logged many more hours of shadowing, spent far more time with patients, and witnessed many more clinical presentations and real-world applications in person.

The academic workload and pressure to make the right connections to secure a match for residency create a certain culture in medical school. It can be a hard environment for anyone feeling out of place, who, despite performing well, is a little "different" or "awkward."

I have personally heard disparaging comments about "awkward" students in terms of their ability to match for residency. But I believe "awkward" students have gifts to bring to the medical profession that perhaps other students do not, and they should not be prevented from advancing in their careers. Future doctors should be *kind* instead of participating in *awkward-phobi*a.

TIME IS FINITE, DEMANDS ARE NOT

Unfortunately, the workload and pace of medical school make it difficult for those students who have the most demands on their time to advocate for themselves.

PARENTS AND CAREGIVERS

Students who have children often find it challenging to juggle medical school with the demands of being a parent. Some parents in medical school even live apart from their children while they complete their studies because of the workload. Their children may live with a spouse or grandparents in another city.

Students who are parents have less time to advocate for themselves, and they may also be prevented from working towards the future they want for *their* children. The only way I have been able to try to address my own needs and speak up for medical students has been by taking time off from school. I am fortunate and grateful that my medical school places a high value on student wellness.

In my second year of medical school, I took 10 months off before returning to finish my studies. It was the best decision I could have made. Looking back, I realize how much I really needed to decompress from school, take care of myself, and spend time with my family after having sacrificed much family time. Also, having the knowledge and ability to raise awareness about issues affecting medical students, I wrote this book.

MINORITY STUDENTS

It's equally important to recognize that minority students generally face a disproportionate burden of issues related to discrimination.[30] They spend more time raising awareness and rectifying such issues both in medical education and in dealing with disparities in healthcare affecting minority groups.

Currently BIPOC (Black, Indigenous, People of Color) and LGBTQ students, as well as those with mental illness or disability, among others, go to great lengths to increase diversity in medical school admissions as well as support and inclusion for such undergraduate and medical students, just as female students did over the course of decades to improve representation of women in medicine. Although medical student numbers show that women are now well represented, only 18 percent of department chairs and deans are women at senior levels of academic medicine.[31]

The percentages of Black, Hispanic/Latino, and Aboriginal doctors across Canada[32] and the United States[33] fall far below the percentages of these racial categories in the general population. The medical profession still has much work to do to address discrimination in medicine and healthcare for many demographically diverse populations, but change is slowly underway.

WORKLOAD WORKAROUNDS

Two ways for medical students to mitigate their workload and possibly have an easier experience in medical school include:

- Learning relevant material in biology, human physiology, anatomy, nursing, or another health profession during their undergraduate studies
- Working in healthcare before attending medical school

Those with strong backgrounds in these areas still find the pace of medical school challenging and still need to study hard for exams. But I have also heard from some medical trainees and physicians—who had prior knowledge or experience—that medical school was the best time of their life and that they were able to coast through.

Another way to ease workloads is for students to take a break at some point during medical training. Some may decide to strengthen their foundation of knowledge by taking relevant coursework or studying on their own. Others take time off for other professional or personal priorities.

Even though I had every reason to take a break from school, it was still a difficult decision to make. A part of me wanted to keep racing forward toward an indeterminate finish line. But administrators and advisors at my school actually urged me to take time off.

I have been told that **no one ever regrets taking a break from medical school**, and I agree that taking a break is well worth considering. I would have missed many special moments with my loved ones if I had not taken a break when I did.

Your child should not have to feel they are at their breaking point in medical school. It is important for them to be proactive and feel supported in efforts to properly rest, rejuvenate, marshal resources, and adequately prepare to finish medical school *well*.

Chances are that your child will know what they need, but may still feel apologetic, guilty, or ashamed about a request or decision to take a break. Give your child the space and support needed to make the right choices.

FINANCIAL BURDENS

Many medical students accumulate debt over the course of their studies, which is another significant stressor. It may impact their career choices if they feel they need to pursue a shorter program and get into the workforce more quickly, instead of picking the career that would be the most fulfilling for them. Many medical students plow through school to achieve their earning potential as quickly as possible, despite any costs to their health or well-being.

Student debt may also prevent students from taking a much-needed break if they don't feel they can afford to take time off. They may be required to make some repayments if they stop their schooling, depending on the conditions of their student loans or lines of credit.

COMMON EXPENSES

Medical students must be prepared to pay for the following:

- Living expenses
- Tuition
- Medical supplies (lab coats, stethoscopes)
- Devices (computers, tablets, smart phones)
- Textbooks
- Online learning resources (software, subscription services for tutorials/videos, practice question banks)
- Application fees (for electives, residency programs)
- Exam fees (for exams required for licensure)
- Professional membership fees
- Travel for interviews, electives, conferences, or other training/work opportunities or requirements (air fare,

ground transportation, accommodations, meals, conference fees, etc.)

- Travel for family visits
- Moving expenses

They are expected to be mobile and go wherever they must to complete their training or work. This often results in separation from their families, partners, or kids.

For interviews, applicants sometimes fly back and forth to the same city multiple times because the interviews for medical schools and residency programs at different institutions are not scheduled back to back.

Because time is at a premium, medical students often take a "pay for whatever it takes to survive" approach to medical school and the costs quickly rack up. They often prioritize saving time instead of money by eating out, ordering take-out, paying for food delivery, driving or using ride-share instead of taking transit, or paying for parking instead of walking from farther away.

They also vary in their spending habits. While some may be frugal or pinch pennies, others may take lavish vacations, wear designer clothing, or drive a nice car.

Many students who are also parents and caregivers end up being severely affected financially. With one parent in medical school and the other parent staying at home to take care of the children, neither has time to earn any income. Meanwhile, they must still support the living expenses of the whole family.

Medical students with a working spouse and children must often pay for childcare or a nanny. When I started medical school, we were also paying for two kids in daycare!

STUDENT DEBT

As a medical student, I have been personally told by representatives at major banks that I may apply for a line of credit well in excess of $300,000. I am fortunate that I have a spouse who is gainfully employed, our living expenses are relatively low, and I didn't have to take on debt to go to medical school.

According to the Association of American Medical Colleges (AAMC), as of 2018, 76 percent of medical students graduate with debt, with a median sum of $200,000.[34] Medical trainees pay off their debt with their earnings once they start practicing as a physician (after completing undergraduate studies, medical school, and residency).

As licensed doctors, depending on what specialty they practice in, they may incur a whole host of overhead costs of up to tens of thousands of dollars each year. They are also usually in an expensive phase of their lives around this time (buying a home and starting a family), which may affect their ability to pay down their debt early on in their careers.

Students who take on any amount of debt can experience significant stress from seeing that negative balance continue to grow over the course of months and years. The sheer amounts that banks are willing to lend medical students are concerning, as is the fact that six-figure debts are considered a normal part of going to medical school and training to perform essential work.

After all, there is still financial risk in taking on significant debt if a medical student has no (or low) income for an extended number of years.

Imagine your child is going to become a franchisee of a donut shop. In order to eventually start turning a profit at this donut shop in five years, your child must borrow and invest $300,000 up front and work hard at the business for the next few years, and thereafter, to also pay down the loan.

Whether you like it or not, from a financial standpoint, this is a fair analogy of the economics of going into medicine. There is risk in opening a donut shop and there is risk in pursuing medicine.[1] The magnitude of the risk and whether it is worth taking varies from person to person.

Within a few years of starting their medical training, some medical students experience what it feels like to be tied in golden handcuffs. They *must* finish their training because they can't see any other options that would allow them to pay back their student debt in a reasonable amount of time.

Yet many medical trainees and physicians—as well as the general public—accept this situation as it is, simply because those who succeed at working as doctors are eventually well compensated.

SAVING MONEY AND PEACE OF MIND

Obviously, if medical students can save both time and money on their biggest expenses such as housing, food, and transportation, they are less likely to accumulate as much debt.

As a parent, you could support your child in this respect by having them stay home with you if you get along well and live close enough to the institution they're attending. This is where having a good relationship with your child pays off financially for them—and perhaps for you, in some cases. However, if living under the same roof is stressful for you or your child and results in daily bickering, complaining, or screaming matches, it probably isn't worth it.

If you teach your kids about managing money and paying off credit card balances in full every month rather than accumulating debt, they may be less likely to rely on debt to fund expenses as an adult. Financial circumstances permitting, they may even choose not to apply for as much credit as they can qualify for as a medical student if they have a habit of staying out of debt.

---

1   This analogy is to illustrate the potential financial risk involved and not to compare healthcare to donuts. Healthcare is a human right; donuts are not!

But **many medical students cannot cover their living expenses during training without student loans and debt**. For these students, looking for everyday savings and managing a budget with the guidance and help of a financial advisor or counselor may be the best way to keep costs under control.

They should also explore what options are available for financial assistance such as scholarships, grants, or bursaries. They should find out whether there are any applicable loan forgiveness programs and make sure they understand the terms and conditions of any loans they take out. There may also be programs available for new physicians to receive assistance in paying back debt in exchange for years of service in some areas.

A last resort that comes with serious consequences, if unable to pay back the student loan debt, may be to file for bankruptcy.

THINKING LONG-TERM

Medical residents have told me that they feel behind in life as they work toward finishing their training—especially compared to others their age who are already working and have houses, cars, and families. If a medical trainee is working to become a doctor mainly for the money, they may resent how long it takes, and be better off pursuing another occupation.

But if they stick with medicine over the long term, their higher earning power has the potential to grow their net worth to eventually exceed that of their peers in other careers. However, they will still need to be careful not to spend too much of it if they're trying to keep up with the lifestyles of other high-income earners.

As a parent, you can work on fostering a healthy relationship with your child and teaching them how to live within their means, both of which contribute to cost savings over the long term.

If your child is doing the best they can to manage their money, it isn't helpful to spend a great deal of time and energy focusing on their balance sheet while they're in medical school.

Becoming a doctor is a long-term pursuit with long-term rewards, requiring significant upfront investments and sacrifices. Your child may not need to worry about the number in red if they are otherwise going in the right direction in life. This is what your child will need to determine over time.

CHAPTER 10:

HEALTH AND SAFETY

Doctors, generally speaking, are known to be exposed to health and safety hazards while working in their profession. As the parent of a potential medical professional, be aware of these issues and be prepared for their risks and impacts.

PSYCHOLOGICAL AND MORAL INJURY

Medical trainees and physicians may experience psychological or moral injuries, whether in their personal lives, over the course of their training, or at work. These can be related to trauma or human rights violations.

TRAUMA

According to the article, "When Physicians Are Traumatized," posted on the Association of American Medical Colleges (AAMC) website in 2019, "nearly 80 percent of doctors have experienced a distressing patient event in the last year, and many go on to suffer from depression, anxiety, and PTSD."[35]

Unexpected patient events (such as patient deaths), medical errors made by physicians and trainees, unintended consequences of medical care, malpractice suits, violence perpetrated against healthcare workers, and even everyday experiences in medicine can deeply affect doctors and medical students, keeping them up at night, and causing them significant stress or even health problems.

Apart from adverse experiences in clinical settings related to patients, medical students are also vulnerable to traumatic stress originating from other sources. For some, the transition into medical school and suddenly taking on the identity of a future physician is a major adjustment and can be disturbing, distressing, and overwhelming, to the extent that it could cause significant stress. This should be treated as seriously as post-partum stress—and access to appropriate care should be made available.

Medical students may also experience interpersonal violence, because they are in a vulnerable, high-stakes position and a massive power differential exists between them and preceptors, doctors, or other people they work with in their medical training.

Historically, some preceptors, and others in positions to provide feedback on the performance of medical students, have abused their power, used physical violence, or otherwise mistreated or undermined students. A recent study of 27,504 medical students in the United States[36] stated that higher prevalence of mistreatment was reported among students identifying as follows:

- female;
- Asian, underrepresented minorities, and multiracial; and
- lesbian, gay, or bisexual.

In some cases, verbal abuse, humiliation, bullying, harassment, or discrimination may not be called violence, but because of the significant power differential between physicians and medical students, and the many stressors that medical students deal with, even seemingly small slights can cause undue stress or harm, and put students at risk of trauma. Such experiences can also contribute to cumulative long-term health consequences.

Doctors and medical students working in emergency departments are often at risk of becoming injured by patients who use violence. Because of high rates of emergency department assaults, in 2019 the American College of Emergency Physicians and the Emergency Nurses Association started an awareness campaign called "No Silence on ED Violence" (#StopEDViolence).

Violence (as a medical and public health issue) and trauma-informed care, are still only emerging areas of medicine. Because of this, I started a student organization in medical school with some of my classmates called Medical Students Against Interpersonal Violence. To date, our members have organized educational events to engage students, physicians, faculty, and community organizations in an ongoing discussion about the role of medical students in addressing violence.

Medical students, just like anyone else, may also experience trauma in their lives due to events outside of medical school, such as the death of a loved one, a relationship breakdown, dating violence or family violence, a motor vehicle accident, serious physical injury or a concussion, or financial loss.

But when stress levels are already high, trauma only makes matters worse and can prevent medical students from performing at their best or even from passing classes.

According to Dr. Albert Wu, MD, MPH, "it's not a matter of if clinicians are going to experience trauma while providing care, but when and how often."[37]

As a medical student or physician, your child will likely experience trauma at some point, and they may need care. You can support and encourage them in accessing any available resources, including helplines for medical students or physicians, or seeing a mental health professional of their choice.

An important tenet of trauma-informed care is to allow people to access and receive treatment on their own time—if, and when they are ready—and not to force anything. People need time to heal, and they need the autonomy to decide what is right for them and when.

To help your child deal with trauma and post-traumatic stress, learn as much about it as you can. You may find that as you learn, you begin to identify and address any trauma from your own life. Healing from your own trauma is an important foundation for helping anyone else with trauma. If necessary, seek out the help of a professional who specializes in dealing with trauma.

Medical students need the support of parents, physicians, and one another so they can advocate for themselves when it comes to addressing violence and trauma. *Self-advocacy is an act of self-care.* When people can speak for themselves, they have far more options than if they feel they can't.

Physicians and parents can only do so much to advocate for students no matter how hard they try. Your child needs their own voice to be heard in order to have real options of help and hope for what it is they seek.

HUMAN RIGHTS VIOLATIONS

Physicians and medical trainees may experience or witness violations against their moral principles or human rights. Such experiences may cause moral distress or injury.

According to Dr. Pamela Wible, MD[38] physicians may be subject to coercion, to either participate in or tolerate:

- Unsafe working conditions;
- Food and water deprivation during long shifts resulting in hypoglycemia, dehydration, and associated symptoms; or
- Dangerous manifestations of sleep deprivation.

A 2019 systematic review entitled, "Resident Physicians Are at Increased Risk for Dangerous Driving after Extended-Duration Work Shifts," concluded that more must be done to prevent occupational and public health risks of driving after such long duration shifts. These include falling asleep at the wheel and motor vehicle crashes.[39]

PREGNANT PHYSICIANS AND MEDICAL STUDENTS

At a conference for Females Working in Emergency Medicine, Dr. Ayesha Khan, MD, of Stanford University and Dr. John Purakal, MD, of Duke University reported that 51 percent of the physicians they surveyed suffered a miscarriage. Two-thirds of those who responded weren't aware of supports or accommodations available to them and most said they wouldn't seek accommodations to avoid being seen as a burden or inadequate. According to Dr. Khan, lack of awareness of the risks of night shifts and long hours to their pregnancy may contribute to low rates of students seeking accommodations.[40]

One systematic review and meta-analysis published in the *American Journal of Obstetrics & Gynecology* found that long hours and night shifts increased risks for miscarriage, preterm delivery, low birthweight, preeclampsia, and hypertension.[41] Even when accommodations are available, physicians who are pregnant feel dissuaded from requesting them because they don't want to be perceived as someone who complains, is high maintenance, or shirks from their work.

Because of this, some physicians and residents are now advocating for protections from night shifts and procedures that involve highly infectious patients for physicians who are pregnant.

SCRUTINY, CENSORSHIP, AND SHAME

Physicians and medical trainees may not feel safe to speak freely on certain topics or in certain contexts because of increased surveillance, scrutiny, and policing of professional and personal activities both from within the profession and from the public.

One example of inappropriate scrutiny and policing of physicians' social media accounts occurred when a group of medical students and doctors searched the social media feeds of young surgeons for "unprofessional" behavior. They wrote an article suggesting that posts about issues like gun control or abortion and photos of drinking alcoholic beverages or wearing bikinis were unprofessional.

When the published article received attention on social media in 2020, it also came to light that the methods used for the study were problematic. Numerous medical doctors responded with photos of themselves in bikinis and swimsuits using the hashtag #MedBikini to oppose the scrutiny of female doctors' attire outside the workplace. In response to the backlash, the journal retracted the article.[42]

Different doctors and medical students have vastly different ideas about what they think is unprofessional, but such incidents recognize that the way physicians define what is "unprofessional" is continuing to evolve.

Freedom to speak out on health-related issues and on wrongdoing in medicine is important for physicians and medical trainees so that they can make improvements to healthcare for the people they serve, and also feel safe as they work.

SUICIDE IN THE MEDICAL PROFESSION

A poster presented at the American Psychiatric Association (APA) meeting in 2018 stated, "The suicide rate among physicians is 28–40 per 100,000; more than double that in the general population."[43] Similarly, the Centers for Disease Control and Prevention (CDC)'s National Occupational Mortality Surveillance (NOMS) catalog indicates that physicians are 2.5 times as likely as other populations to die by suicide. The NOMS data suggests that Black male and Black female physicians are respectively more than 3.5 and 5 times as likely to die by suicide compared to the general population.[44] The CDC "Suicide Rates by Industry and Occupation" data actually reports that healthcare worker suicide rates are lower than the national average, however I believe this may be due to grouping healthcare workers all together rather than reporting physician suicide rates separately.[45]

Based on 2000-14 data from the United States, suicide was the most common cause of death among male resident physicians followed by neoplastic diseases. For female residents, suicide was the second most common cause of death (after neoplastic diseases).[46]

Upon reviewing 1,473 physician and medical student suicides, Pamela Wible, MD, concluded that doctors with access to lethal means, specifically anesthesiologists, are the most likely among physicians to die by suicide.[47]

In "A History of Physician Suicide in America," Rupinder K. Legha, MD, suggests it is concerning that suicide occurs at a higher rate in the medical profession given that physicians, working among other caregivers, should receive adequate care and support. Dr. Legha wrote, "emphases on perfection and discomfort with vulnerability have hindered a comprehensive consideration of physician suicide."[48]

Even though they themselves are proponents of health and human life, and are surrounded by people who care, many doctors do not feel they can talk about their problems.

DIFFICULTIES IN ACCESSING TREATMENT

Physicians do not want to be barred from practicing and seeing patients. However, they may be subject to investigation or punishment by medical boards, licensing bodies, employers, or insurance companies if unwell or found seeking care for mental health.

According to Dr. Pamela Wible, MD, in a keynote speech at Psych Congress 2019, physicians avoid disclosing mental health issues to anyone who may "turn them in" or breach confidentiality. Some avoid filling out invasive forms, obtain care off the grid, or find ways to self-prescribe to protect their own privacy. Fear of being stigmatized or humiliated within a "culture of shame" in the profession may prevent physicians from accessing support.[49]

The 2017 CMA National Physician Health Survey found that "81 percent of physicians and residents surveyed said they were aware of physician health program services available to them, yet only 15 percent had accessed them." One of the reasons given for not accessing available programs was "being ashamed to seek help."[50]

Often, suicide is attributed to mental illness. But according to the CDC, "more than half of people who died by suicide did not have a known mental health condition."[51] When mental illness is cited as the main or only cause of suicide, it is treated as a problem of unhealthy individuals instead of unhealthy social and economic norms or policies.

One particularly heart-wrenching example is that of Dr. Leigh Sundem, who died by suicide after not being accepted to a residency program despite applying for three years. Even though she had achieved numerous scientific publications and presentations, she experienced discrimination for having had a drug addiction as a teen. As an advocate for other people recovering from drug addiction, her career should not have been obstructed.[52]

Everyone has a collective responsibility to dispel the myths about suicide that prevent progress towards real solutions and to also change systemic, structural, or social factors that contribute to suicide.

Suicide is a real risk for students, medical trainees, and physicians. I urge you to learn more about suicide prevention so you can recognize the signs and offer help to your child should it become necessary.

The Appendix at the end of this book lists resources for more information. If you believe your child is at risk at any point, please seek professional guidance and support.

THE CASE FOR HOPE

For decades "resilience" has been a top priority and the go-to solution for human struggles and dealing with adversity.

However, an emphasis on maintaining and increasing personal resilience largely implies we are solely responsible for coping with adversity and taking care of ourselves, which undervalues and exonerates the role of structural and social determinants in the health outcomes of individuals. Meanwhile, exposure to circumstances or events that result in psychological or moral injury, continue to *erode* personal resilience.

Therefore, promoting resilience is not enough. If your child is pursuing medicine, they also need *hope*. Hope can come from the ability to change adverse circumstances and alleviate suffering.

According to a 2020 article in the *American Psychological Association Journal of Traumatology* a hopeful mindset surpassed resilience as a predictor of children flourishing after experiencing trauma.[53] The same could be true for medical trainees.

We all have the potential to create hope for our children, simply by trying. If you are in a position to create positive changes both within and outside of the medical profession, it's up to you to help advocate for and seek answers or solutions that will give hope to the next generation.

Medical students, as a group, have limited experience, ability, and resources especially when their schedules are so demanding. They are often told to keep their heads down and focus on finishing their training before trying to make a difference. Although many physicians "do good" by this and make incredible strides for the profession and for their patients, the fear of retaliation (by more senior administrators, physicians, or coworkers) may never go away.

When I attended a meeting for Doctors for America where many physician activists gathered, one doctor advised students *not* to wait until their training is finished before taking action. Some changes can only be advocated for by medical students themselves.

If your child is interested in addressing an issue, support and encourage them in finding ways to advocate in a respectful, yet effective manner that will be well received by others. Having a voice and options to effect change will give hope, time and time again when things are hard.

ILLNESS, DISABILITY, OR DEATH

Medical students and physicians who have an illness or disability have unique challenges in the profession. They may need to spend more time and money to take care of themselves, treat their illness, or do everyday things that other people don't give a second thought about.

Stressors such as heavy workloads, financial woes, and psychological or moral injury can make medical training and practice more hostile to those with illness or disability, or trigger further health problems.

Trauma and stress contribute to inflammation in the body and put people at risk of developing chronic illnesses and diseases. I have read one too many posts in medical school forums written by former medical students who developed inflammatory conditions during their training.

Bessel van der Kolk, MD, wrote the bestselling book *The Body Keeps the Score* on the topic of trauma. The title says it all. Traumatic stress manifests physiologically in the body.[54]

A 2019 study concluded that medical students have 2.4 times the prevalence of "stage 2" hypertension compared to the general public.[55] Being male and sleeping less than six hours per night were found to increase the likelihood of hypertension.[56]

Last, but most definitely not least, doctors often put their lives and health at risk when they go to work. Doctors and their families can get sick or die from dangerous infectious diseases they encounter.

In the United States, at least three young resident doctors died treating COVID-19 patients in 2020. According to one source, residents had less access to personal protective equipment (PPE) and testing for COVID-19 and were left out of scheduling decisions compared to their more senior counterparts, placing them at greater risk early on in the pandemic.[57]

If you are a parent of a medical student, attempt to advocate for improved occupational health and safety for all doctors and medical trainees.

How? You can:

- Raise awareness on social media.
- Write about it for a blog or newsletter.
- Start a medical student parents' support or advocacy group in your area.
- Support physician/student advocacy or rights initiatives.
- Become politically active and advocate for changes to laws or policies.

One example of a regulatory change supported by parents of medical students was introduced in 2017 when Rep. Keith Frederick presented a bill in Missouri to prevent medical schools from prohibiting or punishing those pursuing studies on mental health issues among medical students.[58]

It doesn't matter that your child is already an adult, medical student, or doctor. If it was anything else impacting their health, the only way forward would be to *do something*.

Yet however beneficial it is to act, at the same time be careful not to embarrass your child with any of your efforts. Many medical trainees and doctors either do not struggle with the same issues as I have described here, accept them as they are, or prefer to turn a blind eye to them, and would oppose or be reluctant to support change, especially if they fear retaliation or negative career consequences.

Being a medical professional comes at a high cost as it stands right now. Support the decisions and choices your child makes for their own health and wellness in the pursuit of meaningful work and help them to advocate for themselves in a respectful manner as an act of self-care. Their life may depend on it.

CHAPTER 11:

THE CHANGING EXTERNAL ENVIRONMENT

Today's changing social, political, and economic landscape is presenting many challenges for the medical profession. Encourage your child to pursue their career plans and make decisions with eyes wide open to these changes: in every problem, there may also be opportunity.

ECONOMICS IN HEALTHCARE

Economic drivers, rather than health protection and promotion, may dictate costs, working conditions, and quality of care. Physicians may experience "overwork and understaffing, a hostile work environment, unsafe working conditions, and failure to provide the resources doctors need to provide safe care,"[59] as described by Alan Card, PhD, MPH, who researches patient and healthcare worker safety and well-being.

It's no wonder that some physicians experience disappointment and disillusionment after finishing their many years of medical training and finding themselves in an assembly-line medicine system. Medical students expect to be able to provide a high standard of care to patients. But after years or even decades of delayed gratification, physicians have at times lamented to me that they were trained for "just a job" in which they are treated as disposable.

Unfortunately, "achievements early in life do not appear to provide an insurance policy against suffering later on,"[60] according to social scientist, Arthur C. Brooks. In 1999, American psychologists Carole and Charles Holahan wrote that people considered gifted at a young age may have "unrealistic expectations about achievement," were less likely to feel they were living up to their potential by middle age, and were also less likely to have good mental health in their eighties.[61]

Interestingly, many doctors do not find a career in medicine to be the most fulfilling. Expectations are a factor, and the inevitability of change is the only thing that is certain. Adapting, innovating, and advocacy for patients and the medical profession are important in the role of the physician.

SHARED TITLES, FUNCTIONS, AND SCOPE OF WORK

One pertinent issue that physicians and medical trainees face is that most people do not know what medical training involves and how people become doctors. Doctors make up a very small percentage of the population, so it's no surprise that many people don't know very much about doctors or medical school.

Today, it's possible to obtain doctorates and other advanced degrees online, which are not the same as MD or DO degrees, but many people do not know the difference. A PhD is a doctor of philosophy and a DNP is a doctor of nursing practice, but neither degree credentials physicians.

The American College of Emergency Physicians has had to create a policy reserving the use of the title "Doctor" in clinical settings for individuals who have completed studies in allopathic or osteopathic medicine.[62]

Additionally, physician assistants, nurse practitioners, and pharmacists can perform many of the same procedures and functions as doctors, such as prescribing medicine. Often, in clinical settings, patients cannot tell the difference between healthcare professionals. They do not always know if they are being seen by a PA (physician assistant), NP (nurse practitioner), MD (doctor of medicine), or DO (doctor of osteopathy).

Sometimes people working alongside medical doctors feel undervalued by comparison. Doctors in some healthcare settings have been replaced by other healthcare professionals who can perform some similar functions as excellent clinicians but at lower costs.

It may be worthwhile for your child to explore other health professions as possible career choices. All professions have their own unique challenges and opportunities.

Since doctors share both their titles and some functions with other professions, in certain aspects of their work, they are unfortunately not well-protected as a profession and oftentimes their many years of robust clinical training may not be economically valued. I must emphasize however, that *only* MDs and DOs are actually trained over the course of (tens of) thousands of clinical hours to practice *as physicians*.

Although controversial, there is also a role for alternative health practitioners, whose therapies are not based in medical science, and people with lived experience who help others based on their stories. Platforms like Mad in America, for example, and patient safety groups raise awareness for those who feel they have been harmed by traditional medicine.

The work of speaking truth, telling personal stories, and creating options outside of traditional medicine are all important. Yet opportunities to collaborate are not realized when different groups disparage, denigrate, or attack one another. It is important to try and work together whenever possible.

During the COVID-19 pandemic, doctors became widely and appreciatively recognized as essential frontline healthcare heroes. But moments of praise are fleeting, so doctors must work diligently to continue developing their profession, while at the same time building bridges and finding common ground with other health professionals, practitioners, and patient safety movements.

GLOBALIZATION

Today, students and workers must compete for jobs against highly-educated candidates globally, and not just against the people in their own small pond. Take a simple phenomenon like the proliferation of the English language. There are more people who have a working proficiency of English around the globe now than ever before in the history of humanity.

The 2019 edition of *Ethnologue*, a credible reference recognized by linguists worldwide, estimates the total number of English speakers at 1.13 billion.[63] An article published by *The Guardian* cited 1.75 billion English speakers—a quarter of the world's population.[64]

As North American medical students and healthcare workers must also compete with English speakers from other parts of the world, competition for admission to medical schools and jobs has increased in English-speaking regions.

Furthermore, for English-speaking students to be able to serve immigrant, migrant, and refugee populations, and to be as mobile in the global job market as people from other countries, they must place some priority on studying foreign languages.

Meanwhile, many jobs are being contracted out to lower-cost workers, wherever they may reside. Work that used to be done in-house for $40/hour is now being done by a third party charging $20/hour or offshored at an even lower cost. Corporations are incentivized to reduce the costs of routine labor, while rewarding those at the top.

When the price that people can charge for labor trends towards $0, workers need to reimagine and adapt their roles in the workplace and in healthcare to these changing circumstances.

AUTOMATION

While some people may believe that "others" are taking their jobs or that jobs must be protected, at the same time, it's important to acknowledge that automation is redefining the very notion of what a job is.

Some argue that automation and artificial intelligence (AI) only change the nature of work, causing new job types to emerge.[65] But others believe intelligent technological advances will cause mass unemployment.[66] Technology and artificial intelligence will likely affect every sector, including healthcare and white-collar knowledge workers.[67]

Like many, when I have a health problem, I generally look it up on the internet, yet *my family doctor is still always helpful and better informed.*

But I cannot say that there won't be major disruptions to healthcare in the near future due to innovation, open access to medical knowledge, requirements for greater transparency, and more capable technology users. Clinics and hospitals are already being acquired by large corporations or closing if they are no longer financially viable, and in some cases, technology makes it possible to care for people remotely (via telehealth for example). Medical students and physicians are relying increasingly on software applications and web-based resources to help them with their work.

With more data and computing power at our fingertips than ever, we will likely see big changes in the decades to come.

This means that doctors cannot *just* do a job. They need to evolve with these new realities. They must also be at the forefront of discussions about where their work intersects with others and with technology, collaborating with all those interested in protecting and promoting human health.

Helping your child to find alignment in who they are, as well as in their work, will serve them over the long term regardless of their chosen career. In order to stay relevant, professionals need to work hard at what they do, and truly be the best. Going that extra mile takes passion, purpose, and the curiosity to discover things that excite them over and over again.

Help your child make a practice out of finding their flow, and they will never *just* do a job.

CHAPTER 12:

ALTERNATE PLANS AND PATHS

We've looked at the information, strategies, and advice for preparing your child to apply to medical school and supporting them through their medical training.

Now, let's tackle the question of what to do if your child *doesn't* get into medical school, or is seriously considering a change to their career plans.

WHAT IF YOUR CHILD DOESN'T GET INTO MEDICAL SCHOOL?

Many students do not get into medical school on their first try. It can take multiple attempts and years of work to build up an impressive portfolio of achievements or experience, and to get better at telling the stories about them.

As a parent, it may be unrealistic to expect a university student to get into medical school upon finishing a bachelor's degree. It is likely that it will take more time, even if your child has a 4.0 GPA and an impressive CV.

Many applicants deal with feelings of shame if they don't get into medical school. Consider what your child would go through. For example, if they apply alongside some of their peers it's likely that not all of them get in. Or perhaps everyone in the family knows they are applying for medical school and has high hopes for them. Many people do not perform optimally when they have such pressures to deal with or if anyone is breathing down their neck.

Your child's career plans do not need to be anyone else's business. Some students don't like being called "premedical," while others don't even tell their parents they're applying to medical school. Students may change their minds about pursuing medicine, or they may claim to have "missed the deadline." Take this as a sign that they are doing what is right *for them*.

You can keep the lines of communication open with your child by not placing unrealistic or unnecessary pressures on them.

Frame medical training or any career plans as a long-term way of life that is challenging and continuously in flux, rather than treating medical school like a get-rich-quick lottery to be won or lost.

Allow your child to retain their autonomy.

For some medical school applicants, the best scenario may be for them to do the opposite of what you advise them to do. Why? Because some people are inclined to blame others for what happens to them, instead of taking responsibility for their choices and actions.

You cannot do much to help a medical school applicant or former applicant who is in a rut of negative-thinking—except to protect yourself from them. In some instances, you may need to give your child time and space to reorient themself after a major setback or failure.

Offer support, and suggest they seek professional help if they're struggling. Also seek professional help for yourself if necessary.

NEXT STEPS

If your child doesn't get into medical school on the first try but could substantially improve upon their GPA or MCAT score, another year or two of schooling, pursuing graduate studies, or retaking the MCAT might be worthwhile.

However, there should be a good reason for doing so other than just trying to raise a score by a matter of percentage points. Perhaps they had a reason for having lower grades or a lower MCAT score, such as not being able to spend enough time studying or a stressful personal situation.

Consider the following questions:

- Has the situation been addressed to improve the odds of your child performing much better this time?
- Regardless of applying to medical school, is your child sufficiently interested in studying a specific subject that going back to school for it makes sense?
- Are they only pursing additional studies to improve their chances of getting into medical school?

Given that GPAs and MCAT scores only account for a portion of admissions criteria at most medical schools, it is worthwhile instead for your child to **pursue unique and challenging experiences that will allow them to stand out and demonstrate their passions and competencies**. But there is no right answer as to what exactly to do to get into medical school.

You or your child may hear people say that you should have something to show for a gap year, like a graduate degree, employment, or some other accomplishment. Such advice is not always grounded in truth unless coming directly from the admissions committee at the medical school where your child is applying. Be wary of the blind leading the blind, and of misguided or conflicting information and ideas. I have met medical students who told me that they basically took "a year off" during a gap year. Why not? It may be the only time they can *rest* above all else over the course of their studies.

I personally stated on my application form that I had young children, had been a stay-at-home mom for a number of years, and that if I didn't get into medical school I would continue staying at home with my kids. The context made part of the difference, because during the same years I was a stay-at-home mom I was also raising awareness about violence—and would have continued to do so.

Whether pursuing further schooling, graduate studies, research, paid work, volunteer work, traveling abroad, or starting a family, *all options are valid*. The right option is the one that is right for your child.

If your child tells you that they need to pursue a certain course of action to get into medical school, such as a specific degree, perhaps suggest that they explore all their options before deciding on a course of action.

If they do need to take specific prerequisite courses, they can often still do a degree in something else if they choose. They should try to select a degree program that will optimize their grades and life experience, although most premedical students have trouble seeing the long-term benefit of doing this because they want to quickly finish their studies with the fewest courses possible.

Encourage your child to find work that is meaningful, purposeful, and enjoyable rather than what they (or you) feel they *should* do. By following their interests, they are more likely to be successful in whatever they pursue over the long term, and to build a truly impressive portfolio. Additionally, their efforts could potentially lead to them building a career in an entirely different field, one that could be more rewarding to them than even medicine.

Someone once asked me, "How do I win an award?" Well, there is no step-by-step "how to win an award" manual. Focusing on winning the award is simply too shortsighted. The same goes for planning towards medical school and dealing with gap years. Asking the question, "How do I get into medical school?" is often not the right question when faced with a situation where you must go above and beyond.

To help your child devise a plan for dealing with gap years or choosing an alternate career, consider asking them these questions:

- What jobs or opportunities can you apply for or undertake with the education and experience you already have?

- What problem would you solve if you could? If you could solve a serious problem that you or someone you love experienced in life, what would it be? If you could solve a problem that would help one billion people, what would it be?

- What did you enjoy doing when you were a little kid? What did you enjoy doing in high school? What hobbies did you have? What groups were you a part of?

- Who are your role models? Who do you admire for their accomplishments?

- What are you good at?

- Is there anything you feel needs to be done right now for any reason? Is there anything you would regret not doing?

- Is there an area in your life that needs to be addressed, such as health, relationships, personal finance?

- Why do you want to be a doctor? What other avenues would allow you to do similar work?

Look for answers beyond money, power, or prestige, because medical trainees do not get to enjoy any of those things for several years.

I personally love the opportunities to work on important and interesting problems in medicine. I have a passion for preventing harm and addressing wellness issues in and out of the profession.

But whether your child wants to help people, perform cutting-edge research, do interesting work, indulge in their fascination with science or another discipline, or be a leader in their field, there are other occupations, opportunities, and areas of study that they can pursue.

Consider the possibility that not getting into medical school—or choosing to leave the profession—could potentially be the best thing to happen to your child.

Explore other options with your child. For example, they could:

- Work at a job, make some money, and get real-world experience so that they have a stronger financial position entering medical school.

- Try working in another healthcare profession to see if they enjoy it.

- Take time to pursue further undergraduate or graduate studies to better prepare for medical school, so that they won't struggle as much when they get there.

- Work on the problem that they feel most passionate about solving, which they wouldn't have time for in medical school, and eventually bring valuable and unique knowledge or experience to the medical profession.

- Try to pursue the work (rather than the career) that interests them, and potentially build a viable or successful career in another area.

- Focus on improving their overall health, get in shape, eat right, and get plenty of rest so that they will be in peak physical condition for whatever career they pursue.

- Have kids earlier in life—if they are in a position to do so—when you (the future grandparents) and they are younger and healthier, instead of putting it off, as many medical trainees or physicians do.

At the end of the day, getting into medical school is not a race. Assume that *the best time for your child to get into medical school is when they actually get in*, whether that's after one, five, or 10 years of trying.

It is never too late, either. I read about a woman who went into medicine and had to leave for personal reasons, but re-applied 25 years later and became a physician in her 50's.[68] If it is meant to happen, it will.

The worst thing that you or your child can do is lament them not getting into medical school and feel that everything in life would be better if only they had got in earlier. You never know what might have happened if your child went to medical school when it wasn't the right time for them: they could have had such a terrible experience that they quit, left due to health problems, or started failing their courses and falling irreparably behind.

That said, when I started medical school, I tried not to kick myself for not applying earlier in life, but I couldn't help it. It was hard being a medical student as a parent with young children. I kept thinking about how much easier it would have been had I been younger. But I also know that if I had gone to medical school earlier in life, I wouldn't have had the maturity, the long-range view, or the life experience to deal with many of the stressors.

I might have quit and perhaps had regrets. I might not have had the adventures that I've had in my life, met my husband, or had my kids. I might not have the people in my life who I treasure more than anything. I will never know.

I hope you can begin to appreciate that not getting into medical school, postponing it, or quitting medicine are not failures. Life is seldom linear, and every experience makes us wiser for the next one, whatever it may be.

JOB PROSPECTS

Of course, if your child is considering medical school, future work is something they need to think about.

In 2019, news channels reported that, "Almost half of all Americans work in low-wage jobs," paying median hourly wages of $10.22 or median annual wages of $18,000 for workers ages 18–64.[69] Many jobs have since disappeared and we have yet to see if new jobs will emerge to replace them.

College graduates have higher rates of unemployment and underemployment than in the past.[70]

If jobs themselves become increasingly scarce, how do we, as parents, help our kids cope with this situation? If your child would love to work at something to the extent that they are willing and able to risk being unemployed for it, they should pursue it. But if employment is a high priority, they should pick an area where they expect employment prospects to be stable.

I've mentioned that applicants can get into medical school by studying something they love. But there is a caveat. They should love working at it so much that they will master or advance the work regardless of whether they can get a job in it.

For example, if a child loves studying biology, but is not willing to work at something related to biology if they remain unemployed at the end of their studies, doing something else that they love or that has better job prospects may be a better plan.

Many factors affect physician job availability, including regulatory and policy changes, workforce demographics, or surging numbers of medical students being trained by medical schools. In the year that your child becomes a full-fledged licensed doctor, there could be either an abundance or shortage of jobs in their specialty.

Some doctors cannot find a job where they want to live and must move elsewhere to practice in their chosen discipline. Many doctors obtain employment in a role that would not have been their first choice. Compromises are sometimes necessary to live in a certain location or to practice at all.

As in every other field, medicine is subject to the laws of supply and demand. This should go without saying, however doctors do sometimes find themselves unpleasantly surprised when reality doesn't match expectations.

Although many practicing physicians report being satisfied in their jobs, medical trainees and physicians must be increasingly flexible and adaptable because jobs are never guaranteed, even in medicine. Even doctors can lose their jobs. This includes residency positions for those who have not even finished their training. Doctors can lose their license to practice, be subject to malpractice suits, or get fired or laid off.

Medical students should expect that "frequent training and new skill acquisition will be required to adapt to the rapid pace of change imposed by emerging digital technologies," according to a Task Force on AI and Emerging Digital Technologies commissioned by the Royal College of Physicians and Surgeons of Canada.[71]

Your child may find that they need to consider other specialties or working in rural or remote areas where there are physician shortages. Pursuing a different healthcare profession or a nonclinical career may also be options.

Medical graduates are already working in entry- to executive-level jobs, careers, and businesses in sectors as diverse as technology and innovation, financial services, government, media, non-profit, and healthcare (of course). As greater numbers of medical doctors pursue nonclinical careers, more resources have become available including articles and even entire books on nonclinical careers for physicians. These may be helpful for your child to peruse.

You may also wish to consider exploring ways to equip your child with the skills to develop, master, and market their own work as an entrepreneur. The next generation of workers will need to invent and reinvent themselves like no other.

CHAPTER 13:

A PARENT'S PARADOX

Current trends create many interesting and complex modern-day challenges for our generation and that of our children, especially with respect to health and healthcare:

- Economic drivers (as opposed to health or wellness) often influence how we raise our kids and how healthcare systems, governments, and markets operate.

- As people are displaced from their jobs, many have great difficulty or are unable to find meaningful yet gainful work, whether that be a job or an entrepreneurial endeavor.

- Not everyone has access to wealth, income, opportunity, justice, or good health.

- Those who have illness or disability or experience poverty or homelessness are still being left behind.

- We may "raise doctors" whose quality of life continues to be magnitudes better than the populations they are trained to serve.

- Yet we still need to "raise doctors" to promote and protect health and human life, elevate (and not diminish) their work that serves patients, and amplify their patients' voices.

- Too many doctors who have trained for eight to 15–plus years for their profession, are no happier than many people who have far less wealth, income, or responsibility.

- At the same time, many highly qualified applicants do not even get the chance to study in medical school in the first place.

I believe it's imperative to raise our kids to the best of our ability, and to produce people who are fully capable of taking care of and treating other human beings in a medical sense. But it is also important to mitigate and curb the harm caused by the dream of raising or being a doctor, especially if it's not the right career path for your child.

Help your child become successful, but also take a long look at the risks and the downsides faced by their entire generation. Our children's generation will still face the problems of mounting debt, devaluation of labor, harsh working conditions, human rights violations, cyber threats, increasing surveillance, and winner-takes-all economics.

Although progress is being made on all fronts, there is still much work to be done.

Up to a certain point, parents decide what is in their kids' best interests. But there comes a time when it must be the children who best know what they want and need for themselves.

What desires and priorities does your child have for their world? Is there any way that you can help or support them to make the world a better place in their eyes?

As parents, as patients, even as medical professionals, we need to really *hear* our kids, our medical students, our doctors—and, most importantly, *do right*, if we can.

CHAPTER 14:

MOVING FORWARD

Understanding what is required of your child to become a medical student and, eventually, a doctor means knowing what they have to do to get into medical school and what challenges they may have to face or overcome in doing so.

You now have some ideas for how to prepare, support, or help your child on their journey.

Just as importantly, you have some context for decision-making and helping your child to determine whether pursuing medicine is the right fit for them. Your child's preferences and circumstances, and what else is happening in the world, are all important factors not to be overlooked or ignored.

Even as I write this book, the world is changing in unprecedented ways, creating uncertainty about the future. Global trends are eliminating jobs in some places and sectors, and people of all ages and backgrounds are migrating to where there is still work. The impetus to do things better, faster, and at a lower cost is impacting medicine just as it is affecting other domains.

There will surely be changes to healthcare, the practice of medicine, and medical education, which needs to evolve with emerging opportunities and new realities.

Being a doctor for the next 30 years will not be the same as having been a doctor for the past 30 years. We cannot go backwards; things will inevitably change.

I've only briefly covered many difficult topics at the heart of the awkward intersections between being a medical professional and a parent, and I have tried to offer balanced perspectives despite any personal leanings. Perhaps what I have talked about has been thought-provoking and engaged you in the space between understanding and uneasiness.

It is in this space that we get better as parents, medical school applicants, medical trainees, and ultimately people. Much work still needs to be done to address the challenges of this profession. Although the work is hard, it is what makes being a medical professional unique. And there will always be a place for doctors who care about the people they serve.

Becoming a medical student and entering the medical profession has been one of the greatest privileges and experiences of my life. Although a part of me wishes that everyone could experience it for even a short time to understand what it is really like, that certainly doesn't mean that everyone *should*. There are many paths to discovering and doing the work one is meant to do.

Trust your child as they follow their interests, but also remember to look for ways that you can create options and hope. We all need hope, whether to be a good doctor or to raise one, to be the best parent we can be or enable our kids to achieve their true potential. Parenthood and parent-child relationships are not to be taken for granted (let alone raising doctors) so I know you have your work cut out for you, as I do too.

It is only by advancing one step at a time and making changes as needed, that I thrive as the eternal optimist. I believe in medicine, in my kids, and in the next generation of doctors. After all, those who came before me, and raised me up, made it possible for me to write this book for you.

You have everything it takes to be the parent that your child needs. Wherever your parenting journey takes you, and no matter what you do, be confident in your abilities. You are a good parent - as good as the parent of any physician - and I wish much continued success to you.

EPILOGUE

If you have a special student or doctor in your life, please consider taking a moment to let them know how much they mean to you or thank them for the important work they do.

For other work and publications about medical education by the same author, visit RaisingDoctors.com.

APPENDIX:
SUICIDE PREVENTION RESOURCES

CANADA

Canadian Association for Suicide Prevention
suicideprevention.ca

Centre for Suicide Prevention/
Canadian Mental Health Association
www.suicideinfo.ca

Mental Health Commission of Canada
www.mentalhealthcommission.ca

For Medical Professionals in Canada:

Canadian Medical Association
www.cma.ca/provincial-physician-health-program

Well Doc Alberta
www.welldocalberta.org

UNITED STATES

Centers for Disease Control and Prevention
www.cdc.gov/vitalsigns/suicide

National Suicide Prevention Lifeline
suicidepreventionlifeline.org

Physician Health Specialist: Michael F. Myers, MD
www.michaelfmyers.com

Physician Suicide Expert: Pamela Wible, MD
www.idealmedicalcare.org

Film: Do No Harm by Robyn Symon
donoharmfilm.com

ACKNOWLEDGMENTS

Thank you to each and every person who has been a part of shaping this work into its final form and bringing it to fruition. Without your insights, advice, and encouraging feedback, this book would not have been possible.

First and foremost, thank you to my husband for supporting me in this project. Medical school, kids, and writing has been a true juggling act and I am ever grateful to have such a wonderful partner and father for our children.

Thank you to M. and E. for taking the time to read my draft and provide your thoughtful input. You gave me confidence that Raising Doctors would be a helpful and important resource for parents.

Many thanks to the team at Book Launchers. You have made this book so much better than I could have done on my own. I am truly proud of what we have accomplished here.

Finally, thank you to everyone who has also worked laboriously, and with great care, to improve medical school admissions and education for the well-being of applicants, students, and future physicians.

REFERENCES

1   "Table 1: Applicants, Matriculants, Enrollment, and Graduates of
    U.S. Medical Schools, 2010-2011 through 2019-2020," Association of
    American Medical Colleges, November 5, 2019, https://www.aamc.org/
    system/files/2019-11/2019_FACTS_Table_1_0.pdf.

2   "Future MD Canada," The Association of Faculties of Medicine of
    Canada, accessed September 21, 2020, https://afmc.ca/en/learners/
    future-md-canada.

3   Dale Okorodudu, How to Raise a Doctor: Wisdom from Parents Who
    Did It! (Franklin, TN: Clovercroft Publishing, 2018).

4   "Table 1. "MCAT and GPAs for Applicants and Matriculants to U.S.
    Medical Schools by Primary Undergraduate Major, 2019-2020,"
    Association of American Medical Colleges, October 16, 2019, https://
    www.aamc.org/system/files/2019-10/2019_FACTS_Table_A-17.pdf.

5   Keisa Bennett et al., "Closing the Gap: Finding and Encouraging
    Physicians Who Will Care for the Underserved," AMA Journal
    of Ethics 11, no. 5 (2009): 390–98, https://doi.org/10.1001
    virtualmentor.2009.11.5.pfor1-0905.

6   Kristen Bialik and Richard Fry, "Millennial life: How young adulthood
    today compares with prior generations," Pew Research Center, February
    14, 2019, https://www.pewsocialtrends.org/essay/millennial-life-how-
    young-adulthood-today-compares-with-prior-generations/.

7   Alecs Chochinov, "CAEP, COVID-19 AND OUR 2020 CONFERENCE,"
    Canadian Association of Emergency Physicians, March 20, 2020,
    https://caep.ca/wp-content/uploads/2020/03/Presidents-Message-
    AC2-March-19-1-signed-FINAL-v1-letterhead.pdf.

8   Decca Aitkenhead, "Panic, chronic anxiety and burnout: doctors
    at breaking point," The Guardian, March 10, 2018, https://www.

theguardian.com/society/2018/mar/10/panic-chronic-anxiety-burnout-doctors-breaking-point.

9   Richard K. Reznick et al, "Task Force Report on Artificial Intelligence and Emerging Digital Technologies," Royal College of Physicians and Surgeons of Canada, February 2020, http://www.royalcollege.ca/rcsite/documents/health-policy/rc-ai-task-force-e.pdf.

10 Kirsten E. Kirby and William M. Kirby, Your White Coat Is Waiting: Vital Advice for Pre-Meds (Boston: Kirby Career Advising, 2019).

11 "Press Release: Thousands of Medical Students and Graduates Celebrate NRMP Match Results," The Match, March 20, 2020, https://www.nrmp.org/2020-press-release-thousands-resident-physician-applicants-celebrate-nrmp-match-results/.

12 Basia Okoniewska et al., "Journey of candidates who were unmatched in the Canadian Residency Matching Service (CaRMS): A phenomenological study," Canadian Medical Education Journal 11, no. 3 (2020), https://doi.org/10.36834/cmej.69318.

13 "2018 National Resident Survey," Resident Doctors of Canada, 2018, https://residentdoctors.ca/wp-content/uploads/2018/10/National-Resident-Survey-2018-R8.pdf.

14 Caroline Mercer, "How work hours affect medical resident performance and wellness," Canadian Medical Association Journal 191, no. 39 (2019), https://www.cmaj.ca/content/191/39/E1086.

15 Carol K. Kane, "Policy Research Perspectives: Updated Data on Physician Practice Arrangements: For the First Time, Fewer Physicians Are Owners Than Employees," American Medical Association, July 2019, https://www.ama-assn.org/system/files/2019-07/prp-fewer-owners-benchmark-survey-2018.pdf.

16 Bennett et al., "Closing the Gap," 390–98.

17 Danielle Ward, Atypical Premed: A Non-Traditional Student's Guide to Applying to Medical School (USA: self-published, 2020).

18 Tabitha Moses, "Medical Students Do Not Owe You Their Trauma," in-Training, July 1, 2020, https://in-training.org/medical-students-do-not-owe-you-their-trauma-20258.

19 Lydia Saad, "U.S. Ethics Ratings Rise for Medical Workers and Teachers," Gallup, December 22, 2020, https://news.gallup.com/poll/328136/ethics-ratings-rise-medical-workers-teachers.aspx.

20 "O*NET Interest Profiler at My Next Move." My Next Move. US Department of Labor, August 18, 2020. https://www.mynextmove.org/explore/ip.

21 Kirsten E. Kirby and William M. Kirby, Your White Coat Is Waiting: Vital Advice for Premeds (Boston: Kirby Career Advising, 2019).

22 Seth Godin, The Dip: The Extraordinary Benefits of Knowing When to Quit (and When to Stick) (New York: Portfolio, 2007).

23 "Sparketype Assessment," Good Life Project, accessed September 21, 2020, http://www.goodlifeproject.com/sparketest.

24 Ben Gilbert, "A congresswoman dared Mark Zuckerberg to spend an hour a day policing the same 'murders, stabbings, suicides, other gruesome, disgusting videos' as Facebook's moderators. He declined," Business Insider, October 23, 2019, https://www.businessinsider.com/mark-zuckerberg-facebook-moderation-congress-2019-10.

25 Alyson Shontell and Allana Aktar, "Bill and Melinda Gates wash dishes together every night, and it symbolizes a feature every strong marriage has," Business Insider, April 24, 2019, https://www.businessinsider.com/bill-melinda-gates-marriage-wash-dishes-relationship-secret-2019-4.

26 Malcolm Gladwell, David and Goliath: Underdogs, Misfits, and the Art of Battling Giants (New York: Little, Brown and Company, 2013).

27 Casey Gwinn, Cheering for the Children: Creating Pathways to HOPE for Children Exposed to Trauma (Tucson, AZ: Wheatmark, 2015).

28 "Kaplan Test Prep Survey: Nearly 40 Percent of Pre-Med Students Say Stress Almost Caused Them to Drop their Plans to Become Doctors," Kaplan, March 4, 2020, https://www.kaptest.com/blog/press/2020/03/04/kaplan-test-prep-survey-nearly-40-percent-of-pre-med-students-say-stress-almost-caused-them-to-drop-their-plans-to-become-doctors/.

29 Ibid.

30 Katherine A. Hill et al., "Assessment of the Prevalence of Medical Student Mistreatment by Sex, Race/Ethnicity, and Sexual Orientation," JAMA Internal Medicine 180, no. 5 (February 24, 2020): 653–65, https://doi.org/10.1001/jamainternmed.2020.0030.

31 "The State of Women in Academic Medicine 2018-2019: Exploring Pathways to Equity," Association of American Medical Colleges, 2020, https://store.aamc.org/the-state-of-women-in-academic-medicine-2018-2019-exploring-pathways-to-equity.html.

32 Rishad Khan et al, "Demographic and socioeconomic characteristics of Canadian medical students: a cross-sectional study," BMC Medical Education 20, no. 151 (2020), https://doi.org/10.1186/s12909-020-02056-x.

33 "Figure 18. Percentage of all active physicians by race/ethnicity, 2018," Association of American Medical Colleges, July 1, 2019, https://www.aamc.org/data-reports/workforce/interactive-data/figure-18-percentage-all-active-physicians-race/ethnicity-2018.

34 Ken Budd, "7 ways to reduce medical school debt," Association of American Medical Colleges, October 9, 2018, https://www.aamc.org/news-insights/7-ways-reduce-medical-school-debt.

35 Amy Paturel, "When Physicians Are Traumatized," Association of American Medical Colleges, August 13, 2019, https://www.aamc.org/news-insights/when-physicians-are-traumatized.

36 Hill et al., "Assessment of the Prevalence of Medical Student Mistreatment," 653–65.

37 Amy Paturel, "When Physicians Are Traumatized." Association of American Medical Colleges, August 13, 2019. https://www.aamc.org/news-insights/when-physicians-are-traumatized.

38 Pamela Wible, "Human Rights Violations in Medicine: A-to-Z Action Guide (Sneak Peak)," Pamela Wible, MD, June 19, 2019, https://www.idealmedicalcare.org/human-rights-violations-in-medicine-a-to-z-action-guide-sneak-peek/.

39 Nicole T. Mak et al, "Resident Physicians are at Increased Risk for Dangerous Driving after Extended-duration Work Shifts: A Systematic Review," Cureus 11, no. 6 (June 5, 2019), https://doi.org/10.7759/cureus.4843.

40 Wendy Glauser, "Is the culture of medicine contributing to miscarriages among female physicians?" CMAJ News, October 15, 2019, http://cmajnews.com/2019/10/15/is-the-culture-of-medicine-contributing-to-miscarriages-among-female-physicians/.

41 Chenxi Cai et al, "The impact of occupational shift work and working hours during pregnancy on health outcomes: a systematic review and meta-analysis," American Journal of Obstetrics & Gynecology 221, no. 6 (July 2, 2019): 563–76, https://doi.org/10.1016/j.ajog.2019.06.051.

42 Julie Ann Sosa, "Editorial: Doubling Down on Diversity in the Wake of the #MedBikini Controversy," World Journal of Surgery, 44, 3587–88, 2020, https://doi.org/10.1007/s00268-020-05751-4.

43 O T'Sarumi et al, "Physician Suicide: A Silent Epidemic," Columbia University Medical Center, accessed September 21, 2020, https://docs.google.com/presentation/d/1-tK2Rt7qy4joyeoam6goH-0hndL1TweGwIdQt-0u1GQ/edit#slide=id.p1.

44 "National Occupational Mortality Surveillance (NOMS): PMR Query System for Occupation (1999, 2003-2004, 2007-2014)," Centers for Disease Control and Prevention, accessed September 22, 2020, https://wwwn.cdc.gov/niosh-noms/occupation2.aspx.

45 "Suicide Rates by Industry and Occupation–National Violent Death Reporting System, 32 States, 2016," Centers for Disease Control and Prevention, accessed September 22, 2020, https://www.cdc.gov/mmwr/volumes/69/wr/mm6903a1.htm#T1.

46 Nicholas A. Yaghmour et al., "Causes of Death of Residents in ACGME-Accredited Programs 2000 Through 2014: Implications for the Learning Environment," Academic Medicine 92, no. 7, 976–83, https://www.doi.org/10.1097/ACM.0000000000001736.

47 Pamela Wible, "What I've learned from 1,474 doctor suicides," Pamela Wible MD, last updated April 10, 2020, https://www.idealmedicalcare.org/ive-learned-547-doctor-suicides/.

48 Rupinder K. Legha, "A History of Physician Suicide in America," Journal of Medical Humanities 33 (August 8, 2012): 219–44, https://doi.org/10.1007/s10912-012-9182-8.

49 Pamela Wible, "Why 'happy' doctors die by suicide . . . (& how to prevent them)," Pamela Wible MD, October 8, 2019, https://www.idealmedicalcare.org/preventing-happy-doctor-suicides/.

50 "CMA National Physician Health Survey: A National Snapshot," Canadian Medical Association, October 2018, https://www.cma.ca/sites/default/files/2018-11/nph-survey-e.pdf.

51 "Suicide rising across the US," Centers for Disease Control and Prevention, accessed September 21, 2020, https://www.cdc.gov/vitalsigns/suicide/index.html.

52 "Leigh Sundem Memorial Scholarship," Georgia Southern University: Center for Addiction Recovery, accessed September 22, 2020, https://jphcoph.georgiasouthern.edu/addiction/leigh-sundem-scholarship/.

53 Ricky T. Munoz et al, "Hope and resilience as distinct contributors to psychological flourishing among childhood trauma survivors," Traumatology 26, no. 2 (2020): 177–84, https://doi.org/10.1037/trm0000224.

54 Bessel Van der Kolk, The Body Keeps the Score: Brain, Mind, and Body in the Healing of Trauma (New York: Penguin Books, 2015).

55 Jacek Bednarz et al., "Abstract P2059: American Medical Students Have a Higher Prevalence of Stage 2 Hypertension Than the General Public: A Cross Sectional Study," Hypertension 74, no. 1 (September 4, 2019), https://doi.org/10.1161/hyp.74.suppl_1.p2059.

56 Caroline Helwick, "Hypertension Rates High Among Medical Students," Medscape, September 9, 2019, https://www.medscape.com/viewarticle/917993.

57 Jacquelyn Corley, "Doctors In Training Are Dying, And We Are Letting Them Down," Forbes, April 5, 2020, https://www.forbes.com/sites/jacquelyncorley/2020/04/05/doctors-in-training-are-dying-and-we-are-letting-them-down/.

58 John Sadler and Lydia Nusbaum, "Medical school mental health bill draws support from citizens, students," the Columbia Missourian, February 1, 2017, https://www.columbiamissourian.com/news/medical-school-mental-health-bill-draws-support-from-citizens-students/article_f7615a8e-e8c9-11e6-9662-43ed448417d5.html.

59 Alan J. Card, "Physician Burnout: Resilience Training Is Only Part of the Solution," The Annals of Family Medicine 16, no. 3 (2018): 267–70, https://doi.org/10.1370/afm.2223.

60 Arthur C. Brooks, "Your Professional Decline Is Coming (Much) Sooner Than You Think," The Atlantic, July 2019, https://www.theatlantic.com/magazine/archive/2019/07/work-peak-professional-decline/590650/.

61 Carole K. Holahan and Charles J. Holahan, "Being Labeled as Gifted, Self-Appraisal, and Psychological Well-Being: A Life Span Developmental Perspective," The International Journal of Aging and Human Development 48, no. 3 (April 1, 1999): 161–73, https://doi.org/10.2190/clu1-deuk-xafb-7hyj.

62 "Use of the Title 'Doctor' in the Clinical Setting," American College of Emergency Physicians, updated February 2020, https://www.acep.org/patient-care/policy-statements/use-of-the-title-doctor-in-the-clinical-setting.

63 "English," Ethnologue, accessed September 22, 2020, https://www. ethnologue.com/language/eng.

64 Nicholas Ostler, "Have we reached peak English in the world?" The Guardian, February 27, 2018, https://amp.theguardian.com/ commentisfree/2018/feb/27/reached-peak-english-britain-china.

65 Steven Globerman, "Technology, Automation and Employment: Will This Time Be Different?" Fraser Institute, 2019, https://www. fraserinstitute.org/sites/default/files/technology-automation-and-employment.pdf.

66 Andy Kessler, "The Robots Are Coming. Welcome Them," the Wall Street Journal, August 22, 2016, https://www.wsj.com/articles/the-robots-are-coming-welcome-them-1471907751.

67 Bob Kocher and Zeke Emanuel, "Will robots replace doctors?" Brookings, March 5, 2019, https://www.brookings.edu/blog/usc-brookings-schaeffer-on-health-policy/2019/03/05/will-robots-replace-doctors/.

68 "Woman details becoming a doctor 25 years after medical school," TODAY, October 14, 2019, https://www.today.com/ video/woman-details-becoming-a-doctor-25-years-after-medical-school-71220805762.

69 Aimee Picchi, "Almost half of all Americans work in low-wage jobs," CBS News, December 2, 2019, https://www.cbsnews.com/news/ minimum-wage-2019-almost-half-of-all-americans-work-in-low-wage-jobs/.

70 Jack Kelly, "Recent College Graduates Have the Highest Unemployment Rate in Decades—Here's Why Universities Are To Blame," Forbes, November 14, 2019, https://www.forbes.com/sites/ jackkelly/2019/11/14/recent-college-graduates-have-the-highest-unemployment-rate-in-decadesheres-why-universities-are-to-blame/.

71 Reznick et al., "Task Force Report on Artificial Intelligence."

CPSIA information can be obtained
at www.ICGtesting.com
Printed in the USA
FSHW020320030221
78091FS